Praise for *Inferno*

Shortlisted for the *Sunday Times*/University of Warwick Young Writer of the Year award

An *Observer* Book of the Week

A *Guardian* Memoir of the Year 2020

***Harper's Bazaar* 10 Women Who Will Shape What You Watch, See and Read in 2020**

'A brilliantly frightening memoir about Cho's two weeks on the psychiatric ward, elegantly interwoven with tales from her past' Lara Feigel, *Guardian*

'This book is utterly brilliant: poetic, truthful, frightening, clever. I held my breath at both the power of the prose and the writer's unflinching honesty' Christie Watson, author of *The Language of Kindness*

'In honest and intricate detail, *Inferno* traverses between past traumas and present-day experiences' *Evening Standard*

'Veers away from being a heart-warming tale of riumph over trauma; it lays out, with frightening clarity, the spiralling pressures of new motherhood and he unvarnished reality of mental breakdown' *Guardian,* Best Memoirs of 2020

'Feels like an important piece of reportage about the condition as well as a gripping personal story' Sebastian Faulks, *Spectator* Books of the Year

'A fierce, brave, glittering book that charts with unflinching honesty the shift from one reality to another and the family ghosts that – without always knowing it – we all carry' Rachel Joyce

'Insightful and shocking' *Stylist* Best Non-fiction Books of 2020

CATHERINE CHO gave birth to her son in 2017. Six months later, she would find herself in an involuntary psych ward, separated from her husband and child. Catherine was diagnosed with a rare form of postpartum psychosis that affects 1–2 in 1000 women.

Catherine works in publishing. Originally from the United States, she has lived in New York and Hong Kong. She currently lives in London with her family.

INFERNO

A Memoir of Motherhood and Madness

CATHERINE CHO

BLOOMSBURY PUBLISHING
LONDON · OXFORD · NEW YORK · NEW DELHI · SYDNEY

BLOOMSBURY PUBLISHING
Bloomsbury Publishing Plc
50 Bedford Square, London, WC1B 3DP, UK
29 Earlsfort Terrace, Dublin 2, Ireland

BLOOMSBURY, BLOOMSBURY PUBLISHING and the Diana
logo are trademarks of Bloomsbury Publishing Plc

First published in Great Britain 2020
This paperback edition published in 2021

ISBN: PB: 978-1-5266-1904-4 EBOOK: 978-1-5266-1907-5

2 4 6 8 10 9 7 5 3 1

Typeset by Newgen KnowledgeWorks Pvt. Ltd., Chennai, India
Printed and bound in Great Britain by CPI Group (UK) Ltd, Croydon CRO 4YY

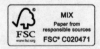

To find out more about our authors and books visit www.bloomsbury.com
and sign up for our newsletters

For James and Cato, the light
in my life

According to Korean tradition, after a baby is born, mother and baby do not leave the house for the first twenty-one days. There are long cords of peppers and charcoal hung in the doorway to ward away guests and evil spirits. At the end of the twenty-one days, a prayer is given over white rice cakes. After 100 days, there is a large celebration, a celebration of survival, with pyramids of fruit and lengths of thread for long life.

When my son was born, I was reminded of this tradition daily by my family and by my in-laws, because we were breaking all the rules. I took a shower after birth, ignoring the week-long rule of no water on the mother's body, and my first meal wasn't the traditional seaweed soup, it was sushi. We opened our doors, let in guests, bundled my son in layers and took him on walks in the falling snow. And then we did a fateful thing: we left our home.

My son was two months old when we embarked from London on an extended trip across the US. I had come up with a plan to use our shared parental leave to do a cross-country tour of family and friends and introduce them to our son. I didn't see why we had to pay attention to Korean traditions – or superstitions, as I thought of them. As Korean Americans born and raised in the US, my husband and I had never paid much attention to the rules, and I had always thought our families didn't either. Except that suddenly, with the birth of a baby, the rules seemed to matter.

We had avoided any evil spirits from California to Virginia, but perhaps we'd just been running away from them, because they found us at last at my in-laws' house in New Jersey. My son was eight days shy of his 100-day celebration when I started to see devils in his eyes.

My husband would take me to the hospital emergency room; by then I would be screaming and tearing off my clothes in the waiting room. I was admitted to the hospital where I spent four days without sleeping.

In desperation the doctors gave me a cocktail of drugs that my body rejected; I still wouldn't sleep.

The decision was made that I should be admitted to a psychiatric ward. I was checked in to an involuntary psych ward in New Jersey, which is where I am now.

It's difficult to know where the story of psychosis begins. Was it the moment I met my son? Or was it decided in the before, something rooted deeper in my fate, generations ago?

My first memory of psychosis is the light.

A bright light. I'm lying on a bed. The room is white, stark and plain. I'm wearing a hospital robe; it feels like paper against my skin. I try to raise my arms, but I can't, there are restraints crossing my body, snaked around my wrists. The restraints are heavy and made of dark cloth, loops that cut into my skin. My hands are clenched. I notice that there are strands of hair in them. There are metal curtains around me; they fold like an accordion.

I try to lift my head, but I can only move it from side to side. I see a man, standing in the corner. He's looking at a clipboard. He has dreadlocks and he's wearing glasses. He looks up and smiles at me gently.

'Hi,' he says. His voice is calm, grave.

'Nmandi,' I say, reading his nametag.

He looks surprised. 'Yes, I'm Nmandi. I'm a nurse here.' He points to his chest.

'Do you remember how you got here?' he asks.

I shake my head. I don't know. I have a vague memory of tearing off my clothes in a hospital waiting room. I remember terror. I can still hear the sounds of screams in my ears. I think they were my own.

My lips are dry, and I try to clear my throat. I find my voice. I want to feel something certain, something to take away the fear. Nmandi is looking at me kindly.

'Nmandi, do you believe in God?' I ask.

He pauses, and he looks thoughtful.

'Fifty–fifty,' he says. 'But I'm OK with that.'

He walks over to me and takes my hand.

'Do you see me?' he asks.

'I do,' I say. And I do see him, in the fullest sense of the word. He's Nmandi, the one who speaks with his hands. Someone who comforts those who mourn and helps those who are afraid. But I also know that he must be the archangel Michael, come to deliver us from the demons.

The rules of time don't exist in a psych ward. Each of us counts the time differently. There are some who count in days, others in weeks and months. And then there are those who don't count the time at all, they've been here for so long. The ones who count in days, they are the ones who pace. I am one of them.

I'm wearing foam slippers, pale blue with smiley faces on them, government issued. I claimed them from the bin, they're now a treasured possession.

I walk past the glass enclosure of doctors, past the TV room where the sound of the 24-hour news cycle is blaring, past the activity room with the conference table, the hallways of resident rooms, to the heavily locked doors, and then back again.

I'm not sure how long I've been here. I think it's a few days. But I count today as day one. The first day that I'm aware of where I am.

In my pocket, I have a folded piece of paper where I've written my truths in purple marker. These are words that I cling to as reality, or at least the reality I hope for. I've repeated the phrases so often I know them like the words of a prayer.

I am alive. *Real.*
I am married to James. *Real.*
James loves me. *Real.*
I have a son. *Real.*

My son is three months old. *Real.*
My husband and son are waiting for me. *Real.*
I have post-partum psychosis. *Real.*

I have post-partum psychosis. I had never understood what it meant to doubt your own sense of reality, to be removed from time. The closest way I can describe it is those moments in dreams where you're not sure if you're awake or still sleeping, but in psychosis, no matter how many times you try, you don't wake up.

The medical definition of psychosis is a mental illness in which an individual has difficulty determining what is real and what is not – it's a loss of objective reality. I had never heard of post-partum psychosis before my own diagnosis. Pregnancy had brought a list of worries – episiotomies, prolapse, pre-eclampsia. I was so preoccupied with the idea of losing my body, it had never occurred to me that I might lose my mind.

When I woke up this morning, my memory was in fragments. I was flooded with glimpses of past versions of my life, real and not real, as though I'd been copy and pasting a paragraph of my life on repeat.

When I reached for my body, I didn't recognise it. My breasts were a network of red angry knots from not breastfeeding, my ribs were protruding and I could feel the edges of my collarbones. I was wearing a hospital robe and my wrists were sore with the marks of restraints. My hair was damp, tied in a strange way, someone else must have tied it. I wasn't wearing a wedding ring. Wasn't I married? I was sure that I was. I remembered a lace dress, roses and ivy in my hands. I tried to remember the song that played at our wedding. But which wedding? I remembered a few, the groom's face was blurred in all of them.

As I pace the hallways, I'm trying to find the molecules of myself, to collect myself in the present, to contain myself.

Any time I try to remember something from before, to hold on to what was certain, I come up against loops, tangles of repeating memories, replaying with different outcomes.

I remember living and dying, again and again, each lifetime of decisions splintered into possibilities.

I go back to my truths. I am Catherine. I am married to James. I have a son.

Counting my footsteps makes me feel reassured. Numbers are certain; they hold a linear logic. It occurs to me that no matter how many steps I take, I will remain constant, in this place.

I try to remember, but I can only recollect moments.

I remember a baby. The curl of a small fist. The feel of a breath against my arm.

I remember a balcony in Hong Kong, counting the seconds while surrounded by the grit of an orange sky, listening to the man pacing inside, hoping he will forget about me and go to sleep.

I remember sitting with my brother under a maple tree, watching the clouds descend, revelling in the silence, waiting for the tornadoes to come.

I remember my first conversation with my husband. His smile. The swirl of bourbon in cut glass.

Mostly, I try to remember who I am.

There are twenty-five of us in the ward, men and women. We aren't allowed shoes, and so we shuffle in socks and slippers. We act as though this is temporary, like travellers at a departures terminal. People come and go, and we wave them off, those who get to exit promise to keep in touch, but we know that they will not. Someone new will appear and join in quietly, and the cycle continues.

There are those who make a fuss, who scream – but we ignore them, it's too much. I've already become part of the routine, it's as though I've always been here. I have trouble remembering anything before; the rhythm of the ward feels innate.

No one talks about their lives outside of this place; we don't acknowledge that there is anything outside this place; instead, we exist separately from reality, obedient to the rules of the ward. We are suspended in time.

We move along to the preordained schedules, waiting in the meds line, waiting to be called to the cafeteria, waiting for lights out.

I can't get used to the smell of the ward. It reminds me of the chlorine of a swimming pool, dank and dark. The walls are beige; there are tiles on the borders like the ones you'd find in a high school. The paint is peeling in places, and there are stains on the walls.

The ward is shaped like a Y, three corridors that intersect in the centre. At the centre of the ward there is a large glass enclosure with a circular desk inside. It is where the doctors and workers stay. The desk faces out onto each side of the ward; it reminds me of the control panel of a spaceship. On either side of the glass enclosure there are two rooms, a television room and activity room, each with a pane of glass so that everyone can see in.

On one side of the glass enclosure is a hallway lined with rooms. This is where the residents sleep. During the day the doors are kept open, and at night they are latched shut. Some of the residents sleep during the day or sit on their beds. There are workers sitting on chairs in the hallway, looking at their phones, standing guard. The workers aren't nurses, as far as I can tell. They wear civilians' clothing. We identify them by their earpieces and clipboards. They don't have lanyards around their necks; I guess it's a choking hazard. Their poses aren't natural, they seem tensed, ready in a moment to jump to attention.

My room is not in this hallway. I am in one of the 24-hour high-security rooms. It's located straight across from the glass enclosure. There is a worker who sits outside my door, making notes on a chart every time I leave.

In the glass enclosure the doctors and workers tap away at computers and talk on phones. They pretend they can't hear us when we tap on the glass.

I am like a zoo animal, except the zoo is inverted, and the cage protects those who belong on the outside. We, the animals, roam.

I wait for the showers to open. I have my arms across my chest, which is sore and so swollen it feels like it's about to bleed. Shara, one of the workers, nods at me. She's hunched over her phone, her hand under her chin.

'Good morning,' I say.

'You're going to shower, baby?' she asks. I nod.

Shara mumbles into her earpiece and makes a note in the chart on her lap, and then she goes back to her phone.

The showers are in closets, doors that open in the middle of the hall next to the television room. There are two of them, side by side with curtains, but really it's meant for one person at a time. I stand by the door uncertainly. I know that Tamyra is going to take the first shower slot, meaning that she'll have the brief window of hot water.

Tamyra swoops in without any greeting. She wears a *Walking Dead* T-shirt that's stretched tight over her belly. She's twenty-one and pregnant with her third child. Tamyra is a returner, residents who are released each week only to return the next. She knows all the nurses and residents by name and presides over them with authority. She is initially suspicious of me, but we make peace when I give her the morning shower slot and let her have my portion of dessert.

I sway from foot to foot while I wait for the showers. Around me, the ward is starting to come to life. In the glass enclosure, I see workers appear from one of the back doors, a door we don't have access to. They turn on computers, unpack papers, open binders. They greet one another, but they don't look at us.

Tamyra steps out of the shower room without looking in my direction; she's wearing shower shoes and a towel wrapped tightly around her hair. She's still wearing the *Walking Dead* T-shirt.

I step into the shower room. The tiles are green; it feels like the showers at the gym, smelling of bleach and mould. I take off my clothes quickly and balance them on the sink; there's nowhere else to put them. I don't have shower shoes, so I stand on folded hand towels. The showers are icy. There's a burst of hot water for a few minutes, and then it pours down cold. I try my best to massage the knots from my breasts, but it's difficult with the cold water. I start to feel like stone.

I quickly dry myself with a small hand towel and shrug on my clothing. I'd found clothing in the shelves next to my bedroom door. Maternity leggings, maternity bras, jumpers that I recognise as my husband's. I'm wearing one of his grey ones now – it's soft, woollen and smells familiar. I tuck cotton wool into my bra so that I don't leak through my clothes. On top of my jumper, I zip up a hoodie. I have my hands in my pockets, so that I can keep hold of the piece of paper with my truths. It makes me feel grounded, a talisman.

I walk back to my room, where I fold my towel and make my bed. The bed linen is grey from being over-washed, and the material is scratchy and thin.

I can't stand being in the room more than a few minutes, it feels so damp. I step outside the room and shut the door behind me. I start to pace the hallways. From the other end of the hall, residents are starting to walk to the cafeteria, it's breakfast.

The cafeteria is at the far end of the main corridor, the farthest from the rooms, next to the heavy double doors that I imagine lead to an exit. Breakfast is at eight each morning. We stand outside the doors until they are unlocked. There are six cafeteria tables lined up in a small room. At the front of the room, two workers pass out trays of hot food. Breakfast is powdered eggs, pancakes, and slivers of bacon.

'Tea or coffee, honey,' Ronnie asks. He's one of the popular workers, with close-cropped hair and a wide smile. Tamyra calls him her man, and he always laughs.

'Coffee,' I say.

I breathe in the coffee. I close my eyes, and for a moment I remember that I have a home, a place away from here. I try to imagine the table, the windows, the view, but all I can think of is the smell of coffee, and then I'm back. Grounded here in the ward.

The cafeteria is quiet; we eat in silence. The windows are frosted over, the tables are crowded in, we have to stand in between them in order to wait in line. The only sounds are the voices of the workers around us. They stand around the tables and in the doorways, their arms crossed. They each have an earpiece dangling from one ear.

Lingering is frowned upon. We have thirty minutes to eat, and we shovel the food into our mouths with flimsy plastic utensils. We file out one by one as we finish. Whoever is last to leave has to stay and help clean up.

Dave is usually the last to finish eating, but he doesn't have to clean because he sits in a wheelchair. Dave is a homeless veteran in his fifties. He has four children. He's black and has a habit of chuckling to himself; he calls himself Chuckles. He spends most of the day wheeling his chair in front of the glass enclosure, waiting for a doctor or worker to acknowledge him. He stands up from his chair whenever he wants to emphasise something, and he often shouts that 'it's a disgrace!' he hasn't been allowed to leave yet. Sometimes he falls from his wheelchair and the workers have to help him sit back in it.

I bring him food from the cafeteria line because there isn't enough room for him to navigate his wheelchair, and he says, 'Thank you, Cathy.' He doesn't look me in the eye when he says this.

Dave calls me a paralegal because he thinks I look smart in my glasses, and whenever I'm writing in my notebook, he nods approvingly, saying, 'Get to work, paralegal!' He likes to shout at any girl in the ward, and he laughs when they flinch.

After breakfast, I stay to clean up anyway. It gives me a sense of normalcy. It keeps me from pacing the hallways for a little while longer. Tamyra looks at me like she thinks I'm a suck-up.

Jeff, a big worker with a beard and a gruff voice, hands me a cloth. I put on a pair of plastic gloves and spray the tables. I pass the jugs of AriZona diet tea and Sunny Delight down the row of tables, and Jeff pours them into remaining gallons to be taken outside to the medication line. Afterwards, I leave, and the doors to the room are locked behind me.

I walk towards the television room. It's where most of the residents spend their time. It's a small room, but there are three couches set up around the perimeter, and a window that's kept ajar. It's also near to the telephone, which makes it a good place to wait for the phone to ring. The TV is small, hung from the ceiling in the corner. It's usually turned to Fox News or episodes of *Law and Order*. The residents perch on the couches; every so often, someone will stand up and start to roam around the halls, and someone else will slip in to take their place. The couches are a dark navy blue, with patches of cotton coming out of the sides. I notice there are deep grooves on the sides of the wood as though someone's been digging their nails into it. In the corner of the room there's a plastic chair where one worker sits.

There's an unspoken rule that the race majority in the room gets to control the remote. Race is all-defining in the ward. Our rooms are divided by race and gender, one arm of the hallway for the Hispanics, one for the blacks, one for the whites. I have to believe it's intentional. I think it's to prevent potential gang violence, but it also makes things simpler. We self-identify by race and age, and most of the residents group themselves by race. The whites sit together at a table, the blacks at another and Hispanics at another. I am 'the Asian one'. It would be offensive, except that it's the most obvious way to be identified, especially if you're not sure of your own identity. It reminds me of the TV show, *Orange is the New Black*, and I feel embarrassed that the only way I can understand this situation is through a Netflix television programme.

I start to see people the way we must appear to each other. Someone with large glasses, someone with big hair, someone with a beard, someone with blue eyes, someone with dark skin. It makes me think of the Guess Who game we played as children. *Does your person wear silly glasses?* It's the way a child sees the world and the people in it. The questions about appearance are innocent, without any bias or nuance, just 'dark skin', 'beard', 'a hat'. I remember my first day of elementary school, a girl walking up to me to introduce herself, 'I'm black, what colour are you? I'm the only black girl in this school.'

I didn't know what colour I was, and it was only the next day, after asking my mother, that I was able to say that I was considered 'yellow'.

I can tell the others are curious about me, the Korean girl who came in on a gurney, stripping her clothes off and shouting that we were in hell, that the demons were coming.

But the rules here are like the rules of prison, you never ask another resident why they are here; even the workers wouldn't ask that.

The TV is turned to Fox News. They're talking about the upcoming Olympic Games.

'Bang bang bang,' one of the residents shouts during a recruitment ad for the army. A worker tells him to be quiet.

Ali moves aside so that I can sit next to him on the couch. Ali was one of the first residents I spoke to. He's the only Middle Eastern resident on the ward. Handsome, lean, he's a pacer like me, he walks with a slow loping stride.

We kept passing each other along the hallways as we paced. We finally stopped where the corners met.

'I see you,' he said. 'Family is difficult.' He gave me a small smile. I smiled back. I didn't ask him why he was here, but in that moment, we nodded to each other.

'Thanks,' I said. 'And yes, they are.'

He smiled.

'I'm not your enemy,' he said.

'Do I have enemies?' I asked. He shrugged and kept walking like he had only happened to stop.

Tamyra is sitting across from us, legs crossed with a comb in her hair.

'How old are you?' Tamyra asks.

'Thirty-one,' I say.

She hoots. 'Thirty-one? We thought you were a student.' Her tone says that I should be old enough to know better.

The worker in the corner looks up. There are two of them in the room, both hunched over their phones. They text about us; they have a chat group where they send messages to one another about the residents. I learn this by watching them. They are careful to cover their phones with their hands and notebooks. Sometimes they laugh, and they talk into their earpieces as though we can't hear what they're saying.

It's 8:45, medicine time. No one announces it, but somehow everyone seems to know when to get in line.

Someone will quietly stand and the rest of us follow. The returners say the names of their meds helpfully to speed along the process: 'lithium, Risperdal, Seroquel'. I don't know the names of my medication, I think I'm the only one who doesn't. The woman scans the bracelet on my wrist. She hands over two small plastic cups; they remind me of the cups for samples of frozen yogurt. I swallow mine obediently, a bitter liquid and two small round pills.

The medicine makes my mouth dry, like it's always full of powder.

Being on the ward feels like being on a deserted island. There are no books, no pens, no paper except for the colouring sheets of blank illustrated drawings that have fantastical creatures on them, centaurs and leopards and griffins.

I have a notebook that I found in my room. I recognised it as one of my husband's treasured ones, a grey one with creamy pages. I know that it is still 2018 because of this notebook. '9 Feb 2018' is written in James' careful hand with the year underlined twice.

When I found the notebook, I'd asked one of the workers if I could have a pen. She'd looked at me blankly.

'May I have a pen?' I mimed writing in my notebook. 'So I can write in my notebook.' I'm not sure why I explained, but I felt like I should.

I waited by her chair, uncertain, and after a few minutes she sighed and walked to the glass enclosure. I saw her talking with one of the other workers; they looked over at me. One of them consulted a dark binder. I tried to look calm, normal, deserving of a pen.

She came back with a black pen.

'Here,' she said reluctantly. 'The doctor said you can have it. But be careful.'

With a pen in my hand I feel slightly less suffocated, like a window has been opened. I write in my notebook whenever I can. The things I remember, the things I know to be true.

The memories come slowly, stacking on top of one another, a picture slowly coming into focus. I feel like I am reconstructing myself from my memories. I am following a thread from the past to the present, and then I will know, I think. I will know how I got here. I will know who I am. And then, maybe I will be able to find a way to leave.

I'm sitting in the activity room, writing in my notebook. The activity room is my favourite place in the ward. The walls are a pale yellow and it has the most light, the windows are frosted over but there's a soft glow that comes from outside. The room is curved, with a large wall of framed glass that faces the glass enclosure. It's usually quiet, but every so often we have music hour, when they blast hip hop through the speakers. There's a circular table in the middle of the room, scattered with markers, crayons and stacks of torn construction paper and half-coloured-in pages of fantastical beasts.

There's a new girl who came in this morning. We heard her shouting in the hallway when they brought her in. Her name is Emma. She stands hesitantly in the doorway, arms crossed. She's Italian American and in her early twenties. She's still dressed in the pyjamas she was wearing when she was brought in from her college dorm. Her pyjamas have PINK stamped on the back. She reminds me of the girls I went to school with, tall, thin, she has a habit of twirling her hair in her hands.

'What's going on here, what's going on. I'm going to sit here. I'm going to sit next to this girl, she seems nice.' She sits next to me and keeps talking, she speaks so quickly she stammers over her words, a monologue without taking any breaths.

Her boyfriend and best friend checked her in. It is exams week.

'I hope they're fucking, I swear otherwise I will never forgive them. I mean, I wish they're fucking, because I can't believe that they did this to me, you know. They better be fucking because then maybe I can forgive them, you know. You know. You know,' she stammers.

'I have to get out of here. Do you know how we get out of here? God. It's a mess. How long have you been here? Do you know how long we have to stay?' She doesn't wait for me to answer. How long have I been here? I don't know. And I realise with a start that I don't know how long I'll have to stay.

'Oh my god, some of these people smell like they haven't showered in weeks. Oh my god.' She is breaking all the rules; some of the residents look at her coldly.

I find myself feeling annoyed, and I realise suddenly that I'm thinking of myself as one of 'these people'.

'Emma,' Will says. He looks up from his colouring. 'You got to relax, girl.' His tone is gentle. Will is a returner. He's been in and out of these buildings since he was five years old. This time around, he's been in the ward for months, but he's being kicked out in a few days. He has a hipster beard, and he's wearing plaid. He would look at home in any cafe in Brooklyn. He's kind, but has a cynical laugh. He doesn't participate in any of the group sessions; he mostly stays in his room.

'The fastest way out of here is to act like you don't want to leave.' He laughs. 'Then they'll get rid of you as fast as possible.'

'You'll be fine,' I say.

'You don't know that,' he snaps at me. And I immediately feel ashamed. It's true, I don't know that. What will happen to him? He doesn't have a car or a job, where will he go? I hear him talking to some of the other residents, he's trying to borrow money for a taxi to pick him up from the ward, otherwise he'll have to walk. To where? He doesn't know, somewhere. The workers feel sorry for Will, I can tell. They smile at him indulgently, and no one says anything when he keeps apples in his pocket or takes a second serving of dessert.

Next to me, Emma is twirling her hair. 'I'm going to go see if they've been able to get a hold of my *avvocato*. Avocado. My avocado.' She marches towards the glass enclosure. Will shakes his head.

'The fastest way out of here is to act like you don't want to leave.' I wonder about Will's comment. How do I leave? I've been waiting, and I become aware that no one has told me whether I will be able to leave, or when. I look over at the glass enclosure, at the people inside, typing at their computers and shuffling through binders. No one official has spoken to me. I have not met with a doctor or a social worker. How long will I be here? I suddenly feel suffocated. I'm caught underwater, and I can only glimpse the surface, but nothing above it.

I try to think of my son. I don't miss him, but his absence feels strange, as though my body knows we are not meant to be separated. I keep reaching for him. I think about the way he used to sleep in my arms, curled, with his cheek pressed against my chest. I remember holding him for hours, staring at his face and trying to memorise it. I should have tried harder, because I can't remember it now.

It is time for group. Not everyone joins. I'm not sure what we're doing, but I follow Tamyra and the others as we wait outside the cafeteria door. The tables have been folded away, leaving only one out. We pull our chairs to sit around the single small table. I sit next to Ali. Dave pulls his wheelchair next to me. We are told that today we're going to be sharing our autobiographies. How we got here.

The monitor is young with a soft voice. He is patient and lets everyone have their turn to speak without interrupting them. He is one of those rare people who actually listens, and it feels like taking a new breath of real air. 'OK, folks, so if you don't already know, you need to have a written autobiography to go from involuntary to voluntary.' He shows us a form; it reminds me of the writing prompts from elementary school with lines to write on. 'Your autobiography will go in your files for the doctor to read. Once you have a chance to read your autobiography, you'll get points to get to level two. If you're already level two, you'll get extra privileges.'

The returners shift uncomfortably; they already know the rules of this game.

They go around and read their autobiographies out loud. We stare at the floor when someone speaks. It's strange to see people start to take on dimension, beyond the identities of race and age and gender.

Tamyra reads hers without emotion. A childhood of neglect. 'I'm a mum,' she says. She says the words easily, and I envy her. She's been in the system her entire life. She wants to work on her temper and be a good mum to her kids. She has two boys and so she's excited that she's going to have a daughter.

There is Mick, a white veteran who was based in West Germany. He slit his wrists in his sister's house. She checked him in because she didn't want to deal with his 'bullshit', and he doesn't blame her. He says he's sarcastic, but that he's got a good heart. He's not been allowed a pen, so he's unable to write his down. 'Does it count if I'm telling my autobiography?' he asks. 'You all won't give me a pen, so does that mean mine won't count?'

Dave sits next to me, twirling a pencil in his hands. His scrawl is like that of a child's, I ask him if he wants me to write while he dictates. He looks at me for a moment, and then says, 'No thanks, Cathy. You concentrate on getting us out of here.'

I think about my autobiography. How did I get here?

How would I begin?

Perhaps I would begin with love.

When I was fifteen, my grandmother kissed my cheek and whispered in my ear, 'May you never find love.' It was a parting gift, like Jacob to his sons, she was trying to protect me.

Koreans believe that happiness can only tempt the fates and that any happiness must be bought with sorrow. As for love, it is thought of as an unfortunate passion, irrational and destructive.

Perhaps they believed this out of necessity, to keep stability in a country torn by war and tragedy. Love was best described to me as the hibiscus in our backyard in Kentucky. Korean roses, they were transplants that burned a tropical sunset colour. They scampered along the fence in a blaze. The petals were delicate and translucent. The stalks were so thick they would tear and shred as they were cut, shaking the entire fence. To try and cut the blooms for the kitchen table was impossible. They were going to stay right there, not move, even as the sun burned them. Their endurance, the same endurance which made the flowers bloom brightly amongst starved bodies after a winter of war and famine, was what led to their downfall. Strength as weakness.

My mother had banished weakness from her world. When my grandmother was pregnant with my mother she had considered an abortion, but a fortune-teller had told her the baby would be a boy. The disappointment of having a fourth daughter in a row meant that my mother was named 'Khet-nam' or 'the end', the harsh 'k' like the sound of a knife. However, by being born at the end, my mother only pushed forward.

I was too weak; I had her features, but softened. My grandmother's warning came too late. I was already fascinated by love and love stories. To me, romantic love seemed essential. I didn't understand how it could be destructive, and I dismissed the warnings as a sign of a repressed culture. I preferred the Western belief in a happy ending.

My mother tried to temper my imagination with stories from Korean mythology and cautionary tales. The heroines were always strong, full of piety and sacrifice. There was Shim Chung who sold herself as a human sacrifice to save her blind father and was rewarded by being reborn in a giant seashell. There was Nong Gae, a beautiful courtesan who danced an invading Japanese general off a cliff. She wore silver rings on each finger and she interlaced her hands around his neck to keep him close, to make sure that he went over the edge with her. She laughed as she danced off the cliff, the trees her witness.

Romantic love did not feature in these stories; it was an afterthought or a deficiency. Love, instead, was a sacrifice. It meant loss, it meant sorrow. Sacrifice, the giving of oneself completely, that was what was required, that was what was expected.

And suffering. As a Korean, I was meant to expect to suffer.

My grandparents escaped North Korea at the onset of the Korean War, leaving behind loved ones that they yearned to see for the rest of their lives. It's a common story: the people who fled, leaving behind parents and children, promising to be reunited, not knowing that the borders would close and all communication would be lost. Instead, they were left to yearn, to wait and hope. Suspended in the waiting. A border – the thirty-eighth parallel – all Koreans know this line of the hemisphere, I used to trace it on the globe as a child. Such a simple line, I'd think, and it had severed so many lives, created such separation.

So for Koreans, to love means to mourn, to know loss. The sweetness of love is tempered by the knowledge that life will return with a bitterness to create balance to the story.

My psychosis, for all its destruction and wrath, was a love story. It was a story of sacrifice; an obsessive search for my husband. I thought I was Beatrice, the one who was assigned to lead my husband through Hell, and that my life was a sacrifice for his.

When my brother and I were children, we would count thunderstorms.

We would see the flash of lightning and begin counting slowly, until we could hear the distant thrum of thunder. We would feel the storm approaching, we could count it into existence and know how many miles away it was, until the storm was upon us and the house and trees would shake in a frenzy of light and sound.

I go back to those breaths, that counting, in moments when I can feel something approaching. Perhaps it relieves the expectation, the dread, perhaps it just reminds me of being a child.

I remember counting the waves of contractions like thunderstorms. I was told to walk to encourage labour. It had been twelve hours already since the doctors had started my induction, and labour wasn't 'progressing'. It was before dawn. My husband and I paced the long hallway; it loomed over us like an aeroplane hangar. I'd count my footsteps until a wave hit me, then I'd pause and bend over and let it come over me. It felt like my body was a clenched fist, and each contraction moved like a wave that I'd have to accept until it subsided. I could feel the start of the next one, as though it was coming from the horizon. I tried to meet each wave without fear, to deliberately give up control.

I could sense that this was beyond my understanding of what my body was capable of. I felt like an instrument, waiting, that deep breath before the first chord of a symphony is played. I was going to be a mother, I thought. I was going to deliver a new life. I couldn't begin to comprehend it.

Emma is dancing. She thinks we're at a party. 'Oh my god, I just want to *baila baila*,' she says. It must be music hour, the workers are playing hip hop over the speakers again. Dave claps his hands, spinning his wheelchair while Emma dances.

'I like your vibe,' Emma says to me after a worker tells her to sit down. She brings markers to colour next to me while I write. Her mouth is moving like she's chewing gum. 'We girls have to stick together.'

Tamyra looks at us, I know Emma doesn't mean to include girls like her.

'I can't believe this place, I swear it's criminal.' Emma's voice lowers to a whisper. 'One of the black guys, he lunged at me!'

She's talking about Darren, a young black guy who came in looking feral. His first night, he screamed in one of the 24-hour monitored rooms. He's a pacer too. He sits next to me at the cafeteria meal times. He is soft-spoken and calls me 'ma'am'.

I feel a sense of protectiveness towards Emma. There's a blind naivety behind her words that sometimes reveals unsettling truths about the ward, whether she's decrying the unfairness of the workers or how no one seems to be taking us seriously. I wonder if she realises how uncomfortable she makes the others feel.

It is Emma who helps me piece together our status. After tapping on the glass enclosure insistently shouting, 'I'm going to call my avocado,' she is handed a stack of paper from one of the workers.

We read the papers together in the activity room. Dave has followed us in his wheelchair, listening as I read out loud for Emma. Both of us have blurred vision, I think it's the medication, and so we read slowly.

'I don't understand,' she says.

But I think I'm starting to. I learn that we are considered involuntary patients and that we are wards of the state.

'Am I involuntary?' she asks.

'Yes,' I say. 'I think we both are.'

I learn that in order to move from involuntary to voluntary, we have to complete a set of levels to prove that we are fit to be released. I then realise why the returners make an effort to keep things polite on the ward. Points are given for friendly behaviour, and with those points you can earn privileges, like leaving the ward for outside recreation time. There isn't much about how we get to leave; it says that it is only when the doctors sign off that we will be allowed to leave.

'Well,' Emma collects the papers. 'I'm getting out of here. Maybe I don't need to wait for an avocado.'

'I like that attitude,' Dave says. He nods at me. 'You're good, paralegal.'

Until the doctors 'sign off'? I wonder what that means.

I look over at Emma, but she's dancing again – twirling around Dave's wheelchair.

In the notebook my husband has given me, I draw a family tree. It takes me a few tries, but I manage it. I put myself in the centre. Catherine. And then a shaky line to James. I put a box around our names and write 'London' above it. We live in London.

Next to James' name, I am hesitant. I know that he has a mother and father. I draw lines to his two brothers, but their faces are blank.

It's easier to draw my side of the family; I remember them as I would have when I was a child. My mother, the most beautiful woman I've ever seen. My father, stern, distant, with broad shoulders and glasses that cover his failing eyes. My brother, Teddy, a boy with dimples and an easy smile.

And then under James' and my names, I write 'Cato' in large letters. Baby. Son. My son.

We chose the name Cato because it meant wisdom. Cato. He was born in November, I know this. Cato has a Korean name as well: Ji-hoon, two syllables, like all Korean names. The first syllable was chosen by James' family, 'Ji' meaning wisdom; 'Hoon' was my parents' choice, meaning contribution to the community. A wish bestowed from both sides of the family.

I write the words I can call myself. I am a daughter. A sister. A wife. Those words come easily. I can remember them.

I stare at the page. And then I write 'mother'. The word looks strange next to the others, it stands separate. All these words, they feel inadequate. How do they encapsulate a person? Who is 'me'? Who am 'I'?

I feel like my memories are floating around me, distracting me from the present. I am still trying to contain myself, to bring myself back to the moment, to bring myself back to this space, to this page. I want to be sure I haven't lost myself, because if I have, then maybe I won't be able to find my way back.

My father was a maths professor. My mother said she chose him because he was the only man who'd ever been able to look her straight in the face. Because of his bad eyesight, she would say laughingly, he was not overwhelmed by her looks. He did not falter or stumble, like the others who found my mother's beauty too intense. My mother always knew that she was beautiful. She held it around her carelessly. She refused to let it be a weakness or a vanity, it was merely factual. Her beauty was alive, wet and breathing; to look at her was a reminder of one's own mortality.

She was all angles, her body stunted from a childhood of malnutrition, and all her energy was pent up in a body too small. She always looked as though she were on the verge of exploding. Her eyes were deeply hooded, brown with a glimmer of grey.

So my father had looked my mother straight in the face and persuaded her to move across the Pacific, with the promise of loyalty and a smile of straight teeth. She noticed his strong jaw and took his quietness to be strength.

While he finished his PhD in the States, he wrote to her every day, long letters of respectful love combined with his views on the world. Her initial appreciation for his devotion became admiration for his convictions. And because he was a maths professor, she knew that things would always be clear, permanent and proven. She would go back to graduate school in her forties to study statistics.

They moved in together in New Jersey – counting pennies to live on my father's graduate student salary. My father took many photos of my mother, and she stands in the Polaroid frames, captured in a moment, her hair in the wind, always looking like she's about to leap. They'd watch films at the graduate school cinema and eat boiled peanuts. They would take the bus into New York City to share cheesecake from Little Italy and walk along the waterfront. They would walk hand in hand and dream about the future. My mother wanted children, my father wasn't so sure.

It would be five years before they decided to have me. By then my father had found a position as a maths professor at a small university in Kentucky. My father liked the geography, the wide hills and limestone cliffs. The land and Southern manners appealed to him. My mother settled in as well, she spent her days watching tapes of BBC drawing-room dramas and learned to speak to the Walmart cashiers in perfect BBC tones when they gaped at her for too long.

My brother Teddy was born three years after me. My mother said she'd planned it that way, but we never knew what that meant. When my mother decided to go back to graduate school, Teddy was left to me most of the time. He was always in the way, but I adored that about him. He was loud and temperamental, and I remember I was the only one who put up with his neediness. I was his Noona, older sister, as he babbled constantly in Korean, 'Noona, Noona,' while he trailed after me.

We played outside under the Kentucky sky. In the winter we built families of snow people, and in the summer we ran around with lanterns of fireflies at dusk. We made mud pies and carved with toy toolsets under the trees until the shadows crept over and pushed us out.

At night we built bonfires and played with ember sticks, tracing curlicue letters of smoke in the dark.

A sensitive child, Teddy cried easily and, it seemed to me, about everything. He cried when it thundered, if ants got in his socks, if the bonfire burned out too quickly, if he didn't have as much watermelon as I did. He crawled into my room at night with a new nightmare and begged me to tell him stories.

I remember our favourite thing was flying a large kite we had got from collecting and sending off coupons on frozen pizza boxes. We lay on the gentle slope of our front yard and I let him tie the string to his thin wrist, but then tied the end again more securely around mine. The kite soared, what seemed to us beyond the clouds. I've yet to see a kite fly like that again. I told Teddy that it was sure to scrape the sky and then we'd see the moon, just keep watching. While I dozed off, he waited and watched, trying not to blink, because I'd promised him.

Inevitably he'd fall asleep or think that he had missed it because he had blinked too much. He never doubted my promises; maybe because I knew what not to promise. I would never promise that he'd be safe from my father's temper.

Every so often, for no special reason on a very ordinary day, my father's temper would overcome him. It served as a punctuation to our childhood, a way to cement memory. Without those outbursts, my father was a shadowy figure, a set of rules. It wasn't until I started going to elementary school that we discovered that the rules we had grown up with were unusual. We knew that we weren't allowed a television or radio: 'I don't like them,' he said. Newspapers were 'written by liars', and we weren't allowed to read books whose authors hadn't been dead for at least fifty years: 'That's how long trash takes to die,' he said. I learned to read with a thick copy of Dickens on my lap, while inside was hidden a fantasy novel or *Anne of Green Gables*, which he still vetoed because it was 'shallow'.

My mother thought these rules were proof of his uniqueness. 'See, he doesn't follow other people,' she would say, and then, 'You know, you two are so lucky. He's the smartest person I've ever met. We should listen to him.' But she still watched her BBC dramas and when he was teaching night classes she played cassette tapes of Korean pop music that she'd brought over with her years ago. My father would scowl if it was still on when he came home. She'd wink at him and sing a few notes, but she always turned it off quickly.

My father kept to himself, he had the whole side of the house that Teddy and I were never allowed into. I'm not sure if this rule was self-imposed or not, but in our minds it was just as forbidden as Bluebeard's Lair or the West Wing in *Beauty and the Beast*. His side of the house was very quiet because he was reading or studying. He never read fiction, although my mother said that he used to, and we knew that he must have from the way he critiqued it. He only read thick textbooks with strange pictures and the occasional Greek texts. Sometimes he banged on the piano, stormy versions of Beethoven's *Moonlight Sonata*. He had taught himself painstakingly in college, but the few pieces in his repertoire were faultless.

He did a lot of calisthenics, endless push-ups with one hand and jumping jacks, breathing heavily. My mother told us that when he was younger he had been somewhat weak and overfed, too bookish – a spoiled family, she said dismissively. But we couldn't imagine that he was ever weak. When my father did come out of his side of the house it was usually to sit with my mother in the kitchen while she studied. He quizzed her, made her laugh, told her jokes. When we saw him this way he looked shy, as though he was humbly seeking attention. But he also looked proud that he had earned it.

To us he was very imposing. When he did speak it sounded like a bark. I've heard rage portrayed as blind, and that's how I would describe the irrationality of his temper and the way he lashed out wildly. But even though it was brutish, my father's anger was a concentrated and calculated one. It was never in my mother's presence, and it was almost always directed at Teddy.

My mother went to Lexington for class twice a week. My father picked us up from school on those days. We were never sure which days to expect him because my mother's schedule varied. We would sit quietly in the back whispering to each other, while he played tapes of Bach. Sometimes he told us to speak up and asked what 'lies' our teachers had told us that day. I think he knew we were impressed by his breadth of knowledge, and he'd make us repeat our conversations at dinner for my mother's benefit, so he could demonstrate the way he'd corrected our minds.

We were picking Teddy up from kindergarten. He was standing on the corner, neatly waiting with a strawberry lollipop in his mouth. It had already stained his mouth and tongue and he had a red ring around his lips. My father asked to examine Teddy's lunchbox. He had overheard my mother's lecture that Teddy needed to remember to save the plastic baggies to reuse them, which he often forgot. I knew this was because Teddy had a secret habit of throwing out the bread, picking at everything in the sandwich middle. He didn't like the way our cheap home-made bread went all spongy. Today he had remembered to save the baggies, but had left the two slices of bread inside. Teddy looked worriedly at me, and I smiled anxiously back at him. My father touched the curling bread with one finger. He laughed, 'Your mother wouldn't be happy.'

We laughed too, relieved. Teddy started chewing on his lollipop. He smacked his stained lips together, and we giggled at the crunching sounds.

'Stop that noise,' my father barked suddenly. 'Finish it.'

Teddy tried to do so quietly, but the candy was too big to swallow. He chewed helplessly.

'You're not finishing it? You waste your lunch but eat candy?'

I wished for the lollipop sound to go away.

'Why can I still hear it? Agh!' my father started screaming. He cursed in English. He reached back and found my brother's hair and pulled as hard as he could. The Honda was speeding on bluegrass, we sat calmly and tried not to breathe. I held out a tissue for my brother to spit out the candy. He did it quietly; it looked like red splinters in my palm.

There was silence, and then again, 'What?! What?' My father's right hand was off the wheel, and it groped behind him. Knowing what was coming, my brother moved his legs for easy access, because at least then the car wouldn't veer. He was a little too late, though. 'Are you dodging me? Eh? Ehhhh?'

No, no, look how easy, we thought. Teddy dangled his scraped legs readily in reach. He blinked at me with big eyes, his scalp red from the tugging, and his shirt a little dishevelled. I sat on my legs so they weren't in the way. By the time we arrived home my father was still seething. He shut the car door without looking at us and slammed into the house.

What happened next was routine. Teddy would wait with me in my room, and we would try to be quiet. My father sat in his West Wing, and we would just wait.

I hated this most, the silence. Sometimes he would call Teddy in. And I would hear the pull and scrape and beat of fists and unclenched slaps. By this time there would be no yelling. Our father would be quiet, concentrated, and very thorough. He was a mathematician, so it was always very rhythmic, sometimes I thought I heard patterns.

By dinnertime, my father would be almost jovial. He'd make sure to serve us seconds to spare my mother having to get up and sit down. He'd make jokes and laugh hysterically, tousling Teddy's hair. My mother would beam, pleased. But we knew. Big eyes stared at plates.

We never said anything to our mother. I think because we hated it even more when she fought with him. And they fought a lot already. Mostly she was the one who started the fights, because she 'couldn't take his silences or his sulking moods anymore'. She would scream and use words in Korean that we didn't know, and words in English that we didn't know that she knew. Her anger was very dramatic. She screamed and threw things, and my father would sit silently and take it. Once when he left the house in the dark, he looked like he was about to sob. This was worse, we thought. Not him leaving, but my mother's drained look and coldness afterward. She would then lecture us on how lucky we were to have him, 'Your father gives up so much for you,' she'd say. And we weren't sure if it was a self-reminder, but she looked angrily at us until we felt ungrateful and undeserving.

These fights always ended well, inevitably with my father coming back and trying to apologise. My mother wouldn't acknowledge him or she would curse indirectly at him for a few more hours, while he waited bashfully. But in the end she would smile, and let him lean against her.

I never understood my father's anger against Teddy. A part of me wondered if it was jealousy. Perhaps he had expectations for Teddy because he was a son, or perhaps it was because Teddy was so clearly our mother's son, with his moon-shaped eyes and high cheekbones. There was something there, a shadow of something, an echo that I couldn't recognise.

It wasn't my father's intention that I would become fascinated by literature and words. I think he hoped that I would turn to numbers, to certainty, but I loved stories. And so I grew up reading Greek mythologies and many of the classics that I was too young for and couldn't really follow.

My father wanted his children to be clean thinkers, unpolluted by commercialism. He had a vision of raising us apart from the world, off the grid, away from any pre-dictated rules except his own.

We learned not to talk about school or pop culture nonsense. It was stifling, but we accepted it because there was no alternative. I'd lie on the hammock under the oak tree and dream, dream of the sky, dream of escape, dream of air.

My father started to lose his eyesight when we were still children. It was devastating for him, a scholar. We tried to be sympathetic, to be less afraid, but it was like trying to learn not to be afraid of a wolf that we are told has no teeth. Teddy and I lived in silence so as not to bother my father, we learned to move as though we were in a library, out of the way; we spoke softly, in whispers, and any words were deliberately chosen. Teddy and I could communicate with just a slight nod of the head, a movement of the hands.

People called Teddy and me foxhole buddies, which was an accurate description. It was just the two of us.

When Teddy quit his job after university and packed a backpack with a tent to travel around the world, I understood. 'I can't explain,' he said to me. 'I just felt like I couldn't breathe.' I knew what he meant. I had felt that feeling of suffocation, the need to walk. I'd often felt the same, staring at the sky, wondering what lay beyond. It was why I'd chosen New York for university. I'd wanted to go somewhere anonymous, a place that was boundless, a place where I wouldn't feel closed in. And sometimes I'd feel that call, especially in the summer, when the wind was blowing through the windows, and the sun was setting between the silver of the buildings. I'd walk until the sun faded and it turned to night, and I'd howl against the wind.

I remember this feeling now as I walk through the ward, trying to shuffle deliberately along the linoleum floor.

Teddy is the first person I call from the ward. There is a payphone in the hallway and I lift the receiver, but there is no dial tone. I hold it uncertainly.

'You have to tell them to turn it on,' Randy says to me. Randy is developmentally disabled, he's one of the residents who don't count their time here. He walks with his hands brushing against the walls, sometimes chuckling to himself, and then, every so often, he steps inside the activity room and screams.

I stand by the glass. Randy helpfully raps on the glass for me. 'Phone's not on,' he shouts. 'And it's time for the phone to come on. About ten minutes ago.' They ignore us, but Randy tells me to go check the phone, and there's now a dial tone.

I don't have any quarters, so I make a reverse-charge call. It takes me several tries to get it right. Teddy's is the first number that I can remember.

'Catherine,' I say to the operator. And then I wait.

'Hello?' My brother's voice is calm, reassuring, familiar. 'Noona?'

I take a deep breath. 'Hi,' I say. I pause, I don't know where to begin.

'I'm glad you called. I didn't know you had access to a phone there.' *There.* Neither of us say where I'm calling from. I have a vague memory of the last time I spoke to him, I was pleading, asking him to turn off the simulation. And he was telling me to be calm, to listen to James.

'Yes, they have a payphone here.'

'How are you?' He seems to falter.

'I'm OK,' I say.

'Have you spoken to James?' James, yes, my husband.

'No,' I say.

'Wait, give me your number, and I'll tell James to call you.' He hangs up quickly and leaves me with the sound of the dial. I feel lost for a moment, and I don't know what to do, so I hang up. I have a feeling of being alone, but I push it aside.

There is no phone call from James. As I soon learn, once the phone is turned on, it is almost constantly in use. We sit in the TV room, waiting expectantly for the phone to ring, and once it does, one of us will rush in our padded socks to answer it. 'Phone!' they shout.

I wait for someone to call my name.

After my mother graduated, we moved to the suburbs of Washington DC in Virginia without much explanation or warning. I was about to start high school, Teddy had just finished fifth grade. My mother had found a job with the federal government in a tall marble building with a view of the Capitol. My father would stay behind in Kentucky. My mother looked regretfully at our backyard, and Teddy mourned his collection of limestone fossils.

We piled our belongings into a car and drove. We moved into a furnished apartment owned by a Russian lady who'd filled her home with china cabinets and orange tapestries. My mother held my father's hand as she drove us to Virginia; there wasn't much talk about what they would do. He visited us every month, sometimes as often as every other weekend. The apartment wasn't large enough for him to have his own area, so he sat silently on the sofa, and we would stay in our rooms.

By the time I went to university, my father's eyesight had stabilised. He could see enough to walk, but he couldn't see faces, and he wasn't able to travel on his own. I never heard him complain, he didn't use a cane, and instead walked carefully holding my mother's hand. He still played the piano, learning each piece note by note, he'd pause to hold the sheet of paper to his face so that he could read the music.

I went to university in New York; I felt strange leaving Teddy behind. My family drove up with me to the dorm.

Teddy carried the boxes of my things; he was much taller than me. He was no longer the sensitive boy who cried about the last piece of watermelon. Instead, I was the one to cry, while he stood stiffly and looked uncertain. When he turned to leave, I saw in his face that used to be my mother's face, the outline and shadow of my father's jaw.

Some summers Teddy would come up to spend weeks with me in the city. He'd appear with a large suitcase and crash at my apartment, sleeping on an air futon at the foot of my bed. During term I called him every day, and we'd talk about his day, about school. My father was spending more time in Virginia, but my brother never talked about him.

Teddy would go to university in Chicago. And somehow, I wasn't surprised when he told me that he would be studying mathematics.

When Teddy decided to walk away from his job and go travelling, he was gone for nearly two years. He sold all his possessions and started to walk. He made his way across Asia, Europe, parts of Africa, and then finally to South America. He hiked mountains and deserts, walking along remote paths. He would call me whenever he had access to a phone, and he always sounded breathless with excitement and wonder.

He took videos of his travels around the world. I'd watch him and think there was something restrained in the way he carried himself, but sometimes I thought I saw a hint of the kid brother I knew. A young boy with dimples who loved to laugh.

When I think of Teddy, I think of us playing in the trees during thunderstorm season, in the yellow calm when the storm is about to hit. We are in the oak tree, the one with the shaky third branch. Teddy sits where the branches begin to spread, the tree's heart. He's wearing green corduroy trousers, the ones I loved and reluctantly handed down. I'm waiting on the first branch, because I know I'll have to help him get down. The Kentucky air smells like bourbon, and we can hear the storm and thunder that's about to come. 'Please don't cry this time,' I tell him. He pretends not to hear me, but nods. We wait as long as we can, shaking in anticipation as the sky changes and the trees around us turn grey. Our mother calls us in, and I help him down so that we can run to the house before the downpour.

I hear one of the workers say that it's been raining. I can see droplets of water caught in her hair. We can't tell what the weather is like. The curtains are always drawn, and the windows are small and frosted over. In the television room, the window that's kept ajar has been shut. I try and remember what it feels like to stand in the rain. To feel something other than fluorescent lighting.

The TV is turned to Olympics coverage all day. It's taking place in Pyeongchang, South Korea, a show of symbolic unity. 'The first time a unified Korea is hosting the Olympics.'

'Koreaaaaaa,' Tamyra says in a slow whisper. She says it with a meaningful tone and looks at me, as though I'm the ambassador for the Olympics. I wonder if I'm being paranoid, but I'm not sure what she's trying to imply. Maybe she knows that I feel like the television is speaking to me. I know I must be imagining it, but the ads feel too accurate, and the Olympic coverage in Korea is the same way. I try to hide my expression when I hear her.

'You have to go to your room again?' she asks with a sly smile. I think she's guessed that I have to go to my room to express milk. 'Mama mama,' she says and laughs.

I keep my face blank and give her a smile before I leave the room. Behind me, I hear the sound of whispering. What are they saying? Is it about me?

I try to breathe. I was born in the year of the tiger; I have to survive. I think of my grandmother, she was born in the year of the tiger like me. We are sixty years apart. According to Koreans, you live a whole life cycle in sixty years. And tigers are guardians in Korean folklore, symbols of courage and strength. I will be OK, I think. I keep my head up when I walk and make sure to look behind me before I enter my room.

The door closes heavily. I glance around to make sure nobody is there, and then step inside the curtain that separates the bathroom. I try to express milk as quickly as possible. It hurts to touch my breasts; they are swollen and red. The strips of cotton wool in my shirt are soaked through, and I throw them away and replace them with new cotton. I try to hurry, I wonder what I would do if someone tried to come in. I don't know why, but the thought makes me feel nauseous. I think only Tamyra has guessed that I have a baby, that I'm a mother, and I want it to stay that way. I straighten my clothing and make sure there aren't any stains when I walk back outside.

I sense that there is tension in the ward. Emma feels it too. 'Gosh it feels hostile,' she says. The television room is occupied by the Hispanics and the whites, the black residents are roaming outside, looking in and talking in low voices amongst themselves.

'Break it up, break it up,' the workers say. Their voices get high-pitched when they start to feel nervous. I notice it. Ali glances at me.

I keep my eyes on my notebook. I press my pen on the paper so hard it tears. Year of the tiger, I think.

We saw my grandmother every summer. We would go to Korea every year to stay at my grandfather's missionary compound. He was my father's father, a minister, and he'd built a church and house on a hill for the missionaries to stay in. The days were long and hot, with the occasional outpouring of rain. There was no thunder or lightning, just the storm and the wet. But for one week of our visit we'd take the train from Seoul down to Busan to visit my mother's mother.

Her apartment was located by the central markets, next to the fish market and clothes shops, under the shadow of a tall mountain. There was the constant noise of the marketplace, the voices from the streets, and the flicker of fluorescent neon lighting.

My grandmother's apartment was small, with bamboo furniture and mother-of-pearl cabinets finished in filigree cranes and cherry blossoms.

She had a fish tank full of tiny fish, guppies and goldfish and fish that gleamed silver. 'It's for good luck,' she said. 'I'm meant to be by the water.'

She'd grown up on an island, 'Dog Island', battered by waves; she'd grown up shaped by the sea. It was the threat of Japanese soldiers that caused my grandmother to get married. The unmarried girls were the unlucky ones; they became comfort women, taken from their homes against their will. My grandmother had married a mainlander. My grandfather was handsome, older, with dark hair and high cheekbones. He was a tailor. During the day he sewed carefully cut suits, at night he would drink too much rice wine and smoke cigarettes with his friends.

They had settled in Busan, a city by the coast, and my grandmother kept fish and planted flowers and looked to the horizon and thought of her island home.

Every visit, we would go to my grandfather's grave, we would visit on a day when there was no rain so the roads would be clear of mud. My grandmother would come with us, quietly holding a bottle of rice wine.

My grandfather's grave was on a hill, where graves were built into the sides of the mountain overlooking the city. My uncle poured the rice wine over the gravestone. We laid out the fruits on a cloth; I remember the colours of the apples and pears tumbling onto the ground. We took off our shoes and bowed, pressing our foreheads down to the earth.

My mother disapproved of superstition, and she didn't let us burn the paper money or incense in the communal offering, but she didn't say anything when my uncle told us to empty our pockets so that the dead wouldn't follow us.

After our offering, we walked down to the car and shook the sand from our shoes. Behind us the graves loomed. We drove to a bakery where we ate red-bean shaved ice, paper parasols floating in the sweet condensed milk. My mother cut the fruit from the grave, long curls of apple and pear falling from her knife, and we listened to the sound of the ocean.

Emma has folded a piece of paper into a fortune-teller, like the ones we used to have at school. Folded peaks of paper with little fortunes written inside. Dave claps his hands, 'Do mine, do mine!' he says, while she tries to remember how to move her hands. I notice that the fortunes inside are blank, she's only coloured them in. 'Pick a colour,' she tells me.

'Blue,' I say.

'Blue, OK.' She pauses. 'B – L – U – E.'

She lifts the piece of blue coloured paper.

She tells me that I will get married and have lots of kids.

'She's already married,' Tamyra says.

'Oh,' Emma says.

I look down at my hands, there's no wedding ring there.

I was twenty-two when I fell in love with the wrong man. It was the summer after I graduated from university. I'd got a job in New York at a corporate law firm, with a marble-floored lobby and a soaring office with floor-to-ceiling glass. I had just moved into a new apartment, I was paying off my student loans and I was living in a city I loved. I knew I was supposed to feel happy, or at least content, but I couldn't help feeling like a fraud.

The finance industry was collapsing, banks were declaring bankruptcy, and in the general hysteria, paperwork kept pouring in. I was working until early dawn every morning, and while I was happy with the overtime pay, the majority of my work was standing by the photocopier, and I felt like I was caught in a never-ending machine.

We were supposed to write hourly summaries of our work in order to bill clients. We had spent several weeks being trained to perfect the art of writing 'succinctly but with description'. I never knew how to write 'five hours of photocopying' in a sufficiently colourful way, and I was always being sent emails requesting that I rewrite them. Keeping track of each hour made me feel anxious, my entire day condensed into neat catalogues of photocopying, collating, redacting. It made me think of the headstones in St John's Cathedral, a graveyard I walked through every morning to go to work. Lives condensed into three chiselled lines.

Drew represented possibility. A dare against what was certain. He was visiting New York from Hong Kong. He'd had a long-term girlfriend before we met. He was said to be a generous friend and a gentleman. All in all, a very 'good guy'. He was a friend of a friend. We met at a party.

I had never been very sure about the description of 'a good guy'; in my experience, the 'good guys' turned out to be the ones you had to be most careful around, but Drew played to the mould very carefully. He was, in his words, a family man who adored his parents more than anything. He told me that he was very loyal, 'a one-woman man' he'd said with a shrug. He had recently broken up with his girlfriend because he felt she was too dependent on him. Drew was convincing in the role of a gentleman. He was charming; he was sweet and sensitive.

He was an easy person to get along with, and everywhere we went he was followed by a posse of friends.

He wanted to introduce me to everyone. It was a whirl of parties and introductions. 'Meet the girl who's changed my life,' he'd say.

They would always smile at me, and say, 'Drew is a really great guy. He's a really good guy, he's a great friend. He's very honest, it's hard to find that nowadays. He's a really good guy.' And I would nod and smile happily, how lucky I was to have met someone so genuine. I never wondered why so many people had to qualify that Drew was a good guy to me – if I had been paying attention, I should have realised that it was a warning.

We spent several months together, and when he left I was convinced that I'd found someone who truly loved me.

Even long distance, he was devoted, phone calls, visits – and each time he begged me to move to Hong Kong. He told me he needed me, that I would be able to find a job. 'I could take care of you,' he said. He seemed to like that thought – 'I want you to need me more.' It was a strange request. He started enlisting his mother's help. His mother was named Leah, a querulous woman who was devoted to him.

'My son loves you so much,' she said. 'He needs you here.'

Hong Kong was a mysterious place and, increasingly, it represented freedom from the traps of New York. I handed in my notice at work and decided to leap.

I arrived in Hong Kong on the day before New Year's Eve. It seemed significant. The entire city was draped in paper and tinsel, there were lights dangling from buildings, figurines of snowmen and silhouettes of dancing candy canes that would light up, several storeys high, blinking in a swarm of red and green.

A year later I was left out on the balcony of our flat. The air was damp from the nearby ocean, and the chill was the kind that settled in your skin. I was on the balcony floor, wearing only a pair of socks – mismatched cartoon animal socks that somehow Drew had forgotten to drag off me before he'd pushed me outside. I was shivering, holding my legs with my back pressed against the glass door. My skin was stuck to the glass, to the bareness of the granite ground, stuck even to the night air.

By that New Year's, I had finally known the truth. There had been many 'incidents' before Leah would tell me he had been this way before. My face was clean, there were no marks on it, but there was a mark on my neck from where he'd held the blunt knife to it, the knife I used to peel apples the way my mother did, in one long, crisp curl. He'd used a belt, he'd paused in the middle to find a thicker one that had a more satisfying snap, and my arm had a bruise from shoulder to elbow and angry welts along my abdomen.

It never started the same way. Unlike my father's anger, Drew's was unpredictable, triggered by anything, by nothing. His rage was superficial, circumstantial. Someone had looked at me for too long, and I liked it. His boss didn't give him a raise, and I wasn't sympathetic. I nagged too much. I didn't understand him. I was being too confrontational. And then, after a while, he stopped justifying it. He must have realised that he didn't need to.

It angered me. I had never thought I would be a 'battered woman', and I didn't think of myself that way. I thought of our relationship as complicated. Drew loved me, he loved me so much, and I was difficult. I didn't know how to make it stop, no matter what I did – if I argued, if I didn't argue, if I fought back, if I let it happen, it didn't seem to matter. And so I stayed with him and hoped, as he promised me each time, that he would change. That he would become a better man.

I enrolled in law school and took classes in the university on the hill. After class, I would take the minibuses that zipped along the mountainsides to tutor expat children. On the weekends we would dress for parties, glittering nights of too much alcohol and stale cigarettes.

That evening, Drew had been unhappy about the way I'd laughed at a joke a friend had made about him. When we came home, he was sullen, I could sense a storm was coming. I counted slowly, waiting for the descent.

Why did I laugh at that joke? I always laughed at him, I never gave him face in front of his friends, he said. Didn't I understand how hard it was for him? How difficult? His rage circled, it gained momentum. And then it started, sharply at first, the opening.

On the balcony, the air glittered with an unknown dust, the sky wasn't dark but a strange milky orange and grey. It was like coloured mist. I wondered if I should jump off the balcony. Silently leaping and turning into this orange night. I couldn't help wincing as I imagined my body naked and sprawling lopsided on the pavement. The cartoon socks. Behind me, through the glass door, I could hear Drew pacing the apartment. And as I feared, his rage hadn't subsided. He pulled me in again.

He was stomping on my face. There was a belt. And then another, and another, they weren't heavy enough, he was shouting. He was stomping on my stomach, stomping on my legs. I could feel his fist on my face, he was straddling me, and punching me again and again and again on the same side of my face. I was lying on the floor, and as I turned my head I could see in the mirror something I didn't recognise. It looked like putty, putty with eyes. It couldn't be right. Was that my face? I wasn't screaming, I wasn't crying. I was just drifting in and out of consciousness.

I fainted.

I saw my parents, I saw my brother, I saw New York streets with the sunset pouring through. I was wearing a linen dress sharing Popsicles at recess with a boy I grew up with. I was catching summer fireflies in my palm, watching them light up, dancing with them like baubles. And then I saw Drew's face again, shaking and shaking me.

Wake up. He was shaking my head so hard it was bumping on the tile floor. He thought he'd killed me and he was panicking.

When I opened my eyes, I thought I saw him feel relief, but then he punched me again.

I passed out.

I went to the hospital. I had a fissure on one cheekbone, and my face was so bruised it looked like it was smeared.

Leah was sobbing when I told her.

'I don't know why he does this,' she said. 'Why, why does he do this?'

And then she told me about the first time she'd confronted him. It was years ago. He and his girlfriend had been out and she had come back with bruises on her arms and legs. Their friends said that Drew had been drinking. Leah said she had confronted him, she hadn't raised her son this way. She screamed, she wept.

His response was to sit on the balcony ledge, looking out to the faint lines of the ocean, his legs over the sides.

He sat there for many minutes, maybe even an hour, she wasn't sure. It was the worst day of her life, she said.

She said she never brought up violence with him again. I thought of all those times that she'd advised me to be kinder, more patient, to be more understanding. This was her son. This was her monster. I knew it was unfair to blame her, but I took all my frustration and directed it at her.

I left one night; it was seven months after the incident on the balcony. I left with only my wallet and phone, dressed in sandals and a thin nightdress. I'd finally realised that Drew did not love me, had never loved me. I wish I could say that it was because of one momentous incident, but it wasn't. I had discovered that Drew was texting his old girlfriend. He'd saved her name under an alias, a boy's name that I didn't recognise. I felt disgusted, cheated. Everything I'd suffered, I'd thought of as a sacrifice, a willing gift to someone in return for the love they gave to me. I'd never thought of the possibility that there was no love here. The certainty I thought I'd found was merely entitlement, and without it I was left with a shadowy, weak pretence of a person. The idea was liberating, but for the first time, I was truly afraid. All these months of violence. What if he killed me now, when I'd finally realised the truth?

I'd tried to break up with him, thinking that he'd be relieved. He'd slapped me hard across the face. It had triggered several days of him not letting me out of the apartment, and I knew that if I wanted to leave, I would have to do it quietly.

'I'm going to go downstairs quickly,' I said pleasantly. I couldn't hear anything except the sound of my heartbeat.

Would it work?

He was lying in bed, his face in shadow, and he shrugged.

I closed the door without looking behind me, and I walked slowly, calmly. Five steps to the lift. I pressed the button. I waited, tensed to hear if the door behind me would open, would he watch me leave? Would he come out?

The lift came at last, and I pressed the button softly and prayed for the doors to close. I walked out of the lobby into the crowd of people still partying on the streets; I kept walking without looking behind me. I kept walking into the crowd, until I was certain no one would follow. I counted my footsteps. One, twenty, fifty, one hundred – how many would it take?

I passed an alleyway I'd been beaten in, I passed the night markets with roast ducks in the window, the shop of the medicine man who served turtle, the bakery with yellow moon egg tarts in the window. I could feel the night air press around me, but I felt nothing. I felt that I'd just walked out of a glass case – I had been able to leave all along, I just hadn't realised it. Everything had shattered around me, and Drew was now like a poison in my lungs, but in order to leave I had to take the infected part with me as well.

The night was running with me.

I kept walking. I was leaving. I was free.

I stayed in Hong Kong to finish my course. During weekends I spent my time searching for air. I walked around the city. I felt like I was being preserved in camphor, the gases and the pollution a haze around me. I felt dull. I couldn't remember what a vibrant sky looked like. I walked the back routes of the city and let myself get lost. I listened to the air, the stiff sound of fabric in the market shops, walked past the men saucing ducks and hanging them glazed, upside down in the windows, contorted around a hook. The shops of wood-block stamps, manuscript paper the size of bedsheets.

I spoke to my mother every morning. I think she had a sense that something was wrong. I told her that Drew and I had broken up, but I didn't tell her why. She wanted to know why I wouldn't come home, but I told her that I wanted to finish my degree, and she didn't question me.

I was drinking too much; I'd drink until I couldn't see anything or feel anything anymore. I drank until I wasn't afraid. Some nights I'd wake up in the hospital with an IV of fluids in my arm, and I'd call a taxi to drive me back to the small apartment I was staying in, hiding from Drew. He never came to find me at my classes, even though I was scared that he would. I thought he had let me go, or maybe he thought I would go back to him, and he was waiting. I didn't know.

I tried my best to disappear.

*

The last time I spoke to Leah she wanted to know where I was living, but I wouldn't give her my address. I knew she would just give it to Drew.

'Please,' she said. 'Drew loves you.'

'I don't think he does,' I said. 'And – I can't be with him anymore.'

'He hits me.' I said it flatly.

She paused. 'I know he's not perfect,' she said. 'But I really think with time, you both can work it out. If you didn't argue so much with him …'

I interrupted, 'I did everything, it never worked. It's just who he is.'

It was as if I had slapped her. How dare I suggest that he would never change? He was her son. She took a deep breath. She said softly, 'I hope you change your mind.'

I wouldn't, I knew this, but I said nothing. There was nothing to say.

On my last week in Hong Kong, a week after term ended, I packed up my belongings and bought a one-way ticket back to my parents' home in Virginia. It felt like a defeat, like I was starting again in a place I thought I'd left behind.

For my last week, I decided to take a hike called the Walk of a Thousand Steps. The route followed a mountainous path along the edge of Hong Kong, you could see the sharp edges of the buildings and the ocean underneath. Each hill would lead to a valley, and then to another hill, curved like a dragon's back. At the midway point of the hike were the Thousand Steps, a series of stone stairs carved into the mountain.

There were no trees, only land, and I wished for wind. The heat was hands pressing on me. I wished that as I walked, my memory would be erased. That each footstep would take me closer to another place, another reality far away from the one I knew.

I wasn't even halfway when I lost count of my steps. I felt like I couldn't breathe, my breath was gone. I couldn't do it. I couldn't finish the climb. Below me I could see the silver-grey of the buildings, sharply outlined like shards of glass, and the ocean, laid out like the sky. It was like looking at an upside-down world.

There, I thought. There was the place of anger and pain. I wasn't able to escape it.

I turned around and descended, back to the polluted air, back to the mist.

Emma's fortune-tellers are all over the activity room. Discarded, half-folded and opened in different colours, but all are blank. No fortunes.

It was a fortune-teller who had told my grandmother that my mother would be a son, ensuring her survival. I imagine the fortune-teller hunched over books, reading numbers and thumbing through calendars, counting the alignment of the stars, and saying, 'Yes, yes, your prayers have been answered. This one will be a son.'

I remember the fortune-seeking boats in Hong Kong. The fortune-seeking boats promised good fortune, all for a generous fee. I learned that it wasn't only for good fortune, but also to absolve sins, and so there were often Triad bosses, dressed in black suits, counting out stacks of cash bills. The sellers waited by the harbour with tubs of silver fish to be released into the ocean. There would be men and women, sometimes grandmothers, leaning over the tubs, pressing money into the sellers' hands. You could tell who had the most sins to absolve – they bought octopus, the most expensive offering.

The sellers would stand quietly and the pilgrims would board the boats with the tubs of fish in their hands. The boat would putter out into the harbour, to around the midway point, and there would be the sounds of chanting echoing over the water.

They would empty the tubs into the ocean, letting the fish swim free, granting life, finding good fortune. The streams of fish fell in waves into the water. There were clever fishermen who waited in small boats to re-catch them. But I loved the idea of absolving sins through granting life. I wondered how they felt, the fortune seekers, looking out to the horizon, wishing their bad luck away.

What would I ask a fortune-teller now? How could I wish my bad luck away? I imagined standing on a boat. I would be facing the harbour, feeling the salt air in my face, watching as streams of silver fish fell into the water, promising absolution.

'You will have good luck today,' Emma tells Dave.

'Damn right,' he says. 'Damn right. Do mine again.'

When I came back to Virginia from Hong Kong, I didn't tell my parents what had happened. My mother embraced me when she picked me up from the airport. I could feel the edges of her body against mine, she felt more fragile than I remembered.

Back in Virginia I felt suspended, out of place. It was as though time had passed in a world outside, but when I'd come back everything was still the same, like it had all been a dream. I decided to play the violin on Sundays at a local retirement home for Alzheimer's patients. 'What a treat,' one of the nurses would say every time I came in.

The home was a beautiful white Victorian building surrounded by a wrap-around veranda that was always empty. The gardens were deserted as well. Inside the home were several floors. On the bottom floor, residents sat in the main living room watching the television.

I went up in the lift, past the coded locks on the doors. I was assigned the Sunshine room, the place for the most advanced patients. The atmosphere in the Sunshine room was chaotic. Nursery rhymes played over the stereo. There was a constant hum of noise, sometimes screaming and shouting, but it felt like there was nowhere for the sound to escape.

Most of the residents sat in the living room, a small carpeted room in the middle of the ward. The residents wouldn't speak to one another; they spoke to the nurses sometimes. Some would sit with dolls on their laps, others with newspapers and magazines, flipping through the pages as though they knew this was what you did with a page.

They would watch me as I rosined my bow and placed the violin under my chin. There was no accompaniment, no announcement of when I should begin. I would just stand and play, and the room would fall into silence. The violin and the songs were transportive. The residents would sit patiently and listen to the simple songs. 'Tennessee Waltz'. 'Somewhere Over the Rainbow'. 'Amazing Grace'. If a song seemed popular, I'd play it again, sometimes three times, it didn't matter that they'd heard it before. Sometimes they would clap, other times they'd forget to.

Some would sing along. One woman knew the words to every song. She would cry when I played 'Danny Boy'. They would all ignore the woman screaming as she pushed her walker.

Playing the violin was transportive for me too. As I played the simple melodies, I would close my eyes and think of childhood days, of fireflies and kites. I was bringing something beautiful into a place that was ugly. It was like I'd found a way to exit time.

Somehow the residents always knew that I was a visitor from the outside world. Even if they weren't sure of who I was, they knew that I was from someplace else. They would take turns talking to me, each wanted some time to ask me questions. They'd wait impatiently for their turn.

One of the women would always touch my hair. 'So long,' she'd say. And then she'd touch her own cropped hair. Another would ask me to spin, while she clapped and pronounced my outfit perfect.

There was a colonel who liked to tell me about his beef-cattle farm, he knew exactly how many of each breed he had and on how many acres. There was another woman who used to sing opera in the great houses. 'I'm here because my daughter needs me to be close by,' she said to me in a confiding tone. 'It's hard, but you have to do what's best for your children.'

There was a woman who always had a handbag on her lap. I don't know what it was filled with, but she clutched it to her side fiercely. 'She's always prepared, ready to go home,' one of the nurses explained. She laughed, but I didn't.

I was drawn to their stories, but mostly I was drawn to this place where time didn't exist. It was a place of memory, of loss, but each treasured memory lasted only for the moment.

'Who is that?' someone would ask, pointing at their reflection in the shiny case of my violin.

They never asked who I was or whether we'd met before; perhaps they were afraid of the answer.

They all told me that today was the day they were going to go home.

I think of us, the residents in this ward, how desperately we want to leave this place. How would it feel to forget, only to remember each time that there was no plan to leave? There are barred doors on each side of the psych ward, like the points of a compass, except that they lead nowhere.

In Virginia I found a job working as a lobbyist on Capitol Hill in a crumbling town house surrounded by white marble buildings. I found riding the Metro into work every day depressing, the brutalist architecture of the Metro stations felt oppressive and harsh, and working under the shadow of the Capitol building I was reminded how much of my work was pushing paper. I worked for a woman with a stretched, Botox-leather face; she would chew ice cubes in an effort not to be hungry. She was a leading fundraiser for one of the political parties, and her mind had a huge capacity for remembering the names of the wealthy and the famous, although she had trouble with mine, even though we saw each other every day.

I moved out of my parents' house and into a small apartment in Clarendon. My room-mate was a federal employee, who I discovered had a drinking problem. It took me all of a week to figure this out; she drank pints of vodka disguised in a colourful plastic cup with lemonade and a straw. We never talked about it, how she never went out or saw any friends, but would sit in front of the television and watch reality TV and drink until she passed out.

I'd escape the apartment at weekends. I didn't have any friends in Washington DC, and so I spent my Saturday afternoons at the arrivals terminal at Reagan National Airport. I'd always loved airports. There was a feeling of possibility, of excitement. The arrivals terminal was my favourite. And so I'd read a book on the Metro and go to the airport to watch the planes fly in. I sat there for hours, watching the people come through, like waves in a stormy sea. I loved watching the reunions. I loved the look of expectation on someone's face before the recognition. The embrace between loved ones.

I'd imagine what their stories were. Who were they? Where had they been? Now they were returning. The reunion seemed so beautiful. It was like the resolution of a discordant chord, a perfect ending, a closing of the loop.

It reminded me of a Korean documentary programme that showed families reuniting from North and South, a select few who had been chosen and allowed to make contact. It was difficult to watch, most of them were sobbing so hard they couldn't speak. Their lives interrupted by separation and uncertainty. 'Brother,' they'd shout. 'Husband', 'Wife', 'My daughter', 'You're alive, you're alive'. 'I've been waiting.'

My mother used to watch this programme and sob. 'Can you imagine?' she'd say. 'Can you imagine?'

I don't know exactly who my grandparents had left behind. They disappeared from the stories, leaving only a faint trace, not even a full memory. I'd hear fragments of their stories over the years, whispers of wives and husbands, children left behind. It was like they existed in a parallel place. Just on the other side of the border, waiting.

'Can you imagine?' my mother had asked me. And I couldn't. How do you live without knowing? With a life interrupted and no resolution? How do you live in a suspended moment? How do you live as a ghost?

We stand in the cafeteria line at twelve o'clock for lunch. There's AriZona diet tea on the tables again. My teeth feel filmy from the diet tea, it tastes metallic, like stale sugar. I've started brushing my teeth every few hours to try to get rid of the taste. We wait in line as Jeff and Ronnie put on gloves to serve food. The meal today is pizza; I get two round discs.

I sit at one of the back tables by the door, next to Darren and Ali.

At the table behind us is the blind girl with flaking skin, her face is bright red and rubbed raw. I try not to stare, but in a room of blurred faces, all I can do is see hers. I can tell the others feel the same way, we make an effort to look away. She stays in her room except for mealtimes. She sits in a wheelchair and has a 24-hour care-giver who sits next to her, wearing blue plastic gloves. She asks her care-giver to tear up her food into small pieces. They have to be bite-size and triangular, she says. She uses her hands to check and make sure they are the right size.

Mick also has a care-giver, he hired one to 'make sure none of you thugs jump me', as he put it. He smiled when he said it, but it sounded a lot like a warning. Darren just snorted, but Emmett, a young athlete with a bright smile, scowled at him.

I learn that having a care-giver is a sign of status. It's an added expense. Mick has one because of his veteran benefits, but I'm not sure why Dave doesn't have one.

Perhaps he didn't have someone to help him fill in the paperwork.

I can't finish my pizza, and Darren gestures to me to ask if he can have mine. I nod. The workers frown. I realise I've broken a rule.

The mood in the cafeteria is tense. I notice that more workers have been gathering in the doorways, watching silently, their earpieces tucked around their necks. Jeff and Ronnie are standing in the front of the cafeteria with their arms crossed, watching us eat. Tamyra accidentally kicks Mick's wheelchair. 'Watch it, welfare queen,' he says. He laughs, but Tamyra doesn't.

Sam, a new kid, starts banging his fists on the table.

'Respect your elders,' Tamyra snaps.

There is a moment when it feels like something's about to break, and I hold my breath and count. One of the workers tells Tamyra to take a walk, and the feeling disappears.

'Cat, phone!' Darren shouts for me. I'm sitting in the activity room, there are markers and crayons scattered around the table. I'm writing in my notebook. I'm trying to remember everyone's names. I cover the paper with my hands, hoping that no one can read over my shoulder. My pen is starting to run out of ink.

I tuck the notebook under my arm and shuffle over to the hallway for the payphone; I feel eyes on me.

'Hello?'

'Hello, Cat?'

The voice is faint, familiar. It's James' voice. I take a deep breath and try to remember. James. He is my husband. This is my husband's voice.

'Hi,' I say.

'I'm so happy to talk to you,' he says. He sounds like he's on the verge of tears.

I want to reassure him, reach out to him, but instead I close my eyes and listen.

He's asking me questions. 'Are you eating OK? Are you sleeping OK? Are people treating you well? They've said that you have your own room, you do right?'

The questions are spilling around me, and I can't focus. I hear his words pouring over me, and all I can concentrate on is his voice. His voice sounds like it's coming from a far distance. Where is he? I remember hearing his voice during my psychosis, it was always there, as though he was just out of reach. I listen.

'I'm going to come visit, OK? I'll be there tomorrow, that's the next visiting session. I came to visit you yesterday, but you were sleeping, so they wouldn't let me see you.'

I feel like my mind is trying to catch up. I hadn't realised that there were visiting hours.

'When are you coming?'

'Tomorrow night at 5:30, I'll be there,' he says.

'Cato is next to me right now. Can you hear him?'

And I hear the sound of a baby cooing.

My breath catches in my throat. I want to weep, but I also can't feel anything, my mind feels like there's a door, opening and closing, opening and closing. Cato.

'We miss you,' James says. He hangs up.

I hang up slowly. I can feel tears caught in my eyes, but they aren't heavy enough to fall. I'll be seeing James tomorrow. I know that I should be excited, but I feel numb. Somewhere there is a spark of emotion, but I can't access it.

When I go back to the activity room, I look again at my family tree. James. Husband.

I met my husband, James, at a wedding in New Jersey. It had been many months since Hong Kong. I was still working in Washington DC as a lobbyist. I was living back at my parents' home; I'd moved out of the apartment with my alcoholic room-mate. It had become untenable. She would drink until she passed out on the floor, her plastic cups rolling around under the couch. I found out that because she had security clearance, she also had access to a gun in the apartment, and that's when I decided to go. I was ready to leave my job as well. I had been trying to figure out the best way to quit without any blowback, and I was almost ready to pull the trigger.

Hong Kong seemed like a scene from someone else's life, although sometimes my cheekbone hurt, and then I'd be reminded of the bruises underneath the surface.

It was a few weeks before the wedding when my friend, the bride, said that I should meet one of the groomsmen. 'He's a professor,' she said. I pictured a serious-looking man with elbow patches on his clothes.

'But he breakdances. I think you guys would get along,' she said. 'He lives in London.'

I learned that James was a Korean-American from New Jersey, he'd lived in Oxford before moving to London, and he was doing research in something sciencey.

I was reluctant, I didn't need to meet another man who lived across an ocean, and I knew Korean-American New Jersey boys, they were a dime a dozen, I thought.

I'd find out later that James initially refused to meet me as well. 'I live in London,' he said. 'I don't do long distance.'

But it was cocktail hour at the wedding, we'd heard the vows, the sun was beginning to set, and the couple was ready for magic hour. One of my friends dragged me over to introduce me to James. I was surprised to see a boy; he was tall with a shaggy haircut and he had a playful smile. He was laughing with a group of people, but I noticed that he held himself differently, like he was standing slightly apart. In his hand was a glass of bourbon, shining in the cut glass.

'Hello,' he said, and he beamed at me like we were friends. His smile was wide and his eyes were kind, I saw myself reflected in them. It felt as though he was throwing a rope to me, like I hadn't realised that I'd been alone at sea, and suddenly there was someone who recognised me. James would tell me that he felt like he was being 'seen' for the first time in his life.

We saw each other.

I don't remember what my friend said to introduce us, but we started to talk. Slowly and then with increasing speed.

We talked about London, about the theatre, about museums. We talked about our childhoods. He told me about being a kid in New Jersey, his culture shock when he moved to Michigan for university. I told him about Kentucky, about my days with Teddy in the backyard.

As we talked, we forgot about the wedding. James almost missed his groomsman duties; he was pulled away just in time. Around us were the lights and whirl of the wedding, I could glimpse the last rays of sunset and hear the sounds of music and dancing. As he left, he turned back towards me and smiled and waved. 'I'll come find you later,' he said.

And I knew that he would. What was it about James? There was something disarming about him. When I had more time to think about it in the days after the wedding, I'd realise that he was the most sincere person I'd ever met. He was completely open, unapologetically himself.

'I'm flying back tomorrow morning,' he said to me when he found me later. Tomorrow morning? I thought. That's no time at all. But he smiled at me, and looked so calm that I tried to ignore the time, counting the hours slowly to make each moment last longer. The wedding passed in stages, the bride's first dance with her father, her waltz with her husband, the courses of chicken and beef, the speeches, cocktails, but we were suspended, caught in the moment we had met.

And because we only had one night, we spent it together talking. I learned about James' vision, his dream to create non-invasive surgery using ultrasound. He told me about his family, a large clan spread across California and New York, their weekly dinners and summers of barbecues and pool parties. I learned that his father was slightly deaf, and I laughed – he was the son of a deaf man, and I was the daughter of a blind man.

'What's your dream?' he asked me.

'I don't have one,' I said. 'But I wish I did.' I wanted some of his certainty, some of his hope and drive for the future. I realised that he was always looking ahead, looking to the future, while I was fascinated by the past, reliving memories again and again. And so, with the future and past together, each hour passed like a dream; we were existing outside of time.

He never mentioned the future to me, although I could tell he was thinking about it. He'd give me an appraising look, as if trying to guess if I was thinking what he was thinking. At one point, he suddenly said to me, 'So, we're really going to do this?'

'What do you mean?' I asked.

'We're going to date. Even though I live in London and you're here.'

I laughed. 'Why not?'

And he laughed too.

James would tell me later that he fell in love with me at first conversation. The room seemed to blur, he said, and all I could see was you. We had good rhythm, he said. And we did – the way we talked, the way the conversation flowed, it was familiar, like the well-known notes of an old song.

The next morning, James flew back to London. He'd given me his email address, his mobile and office phone numbers, his website, and home and office addresses. There would be no excuse, he said. He called me when I landed in London. 'I've been thinking of you,' he said. 'I was thinking of you on my flight back, and I'm thinking of you now.'

He asked me to visit him in London. I agreed to visit a month later after I had quit my job. I'd already promised myself that I would quit, but the trip to London gave me a reason to make sure I kept my promise.

While we waited for my trip, we talked for hours on the phone and on FaceTime. We played questions, where we had to guess the other's answer to a question we posed. What was our favourite part of the day? What did we most look forward to? What was our idea of a perfect date? We planned outings, imagined a list of places we'd go when I was in London. Have ice cream on the Millennium Bridge, visit the Tate Modern, watch a play at the National Theatre, walk through Richmond Park. We treasured each like they were already memories. There was beauty in the waiting.

I packed my bag for six weeks. It was autumn in London. As I boarded, I touched the side of the plane for good luck. I felt a sense of repetition, a recurrence. But it wasn't, was it? This time I was flying across the Atlantic, to someone new.

At the airport, I saw James waiting at the arrivals gate. I tried to think of how we looked to the people around us. All those times I'd sat and watched couples like us reunite, I had never known their stories but I had wondered about them at that moment, the moment of two lives intersecting. I suddenly felt shy and uncertain. What was I doing? Did I even know this guy? I'd only known him for twelve hours, and here I was, we were going to spend six weeks together. He was smiling; his hair was still shaggy. I paused, hesitant, and he stepped forwards to embrace me. When he embraced me, all doubt disappeared.

We stayed in his studio apartment near Hyde Park. James presented me with two notebooks, one for me and one for us to write in together. For our adventures, he said.

London became our playground. We went through our list of dates, savouring each moment that had before been only imaginary. We lounged and drank coffee at cafes, walked hand in hand through Hyde Park, wandered through museums of gilded stone and marble. Each moment felt precious – we knew it was temporary, and so we held on to them.

But throughout, we talked. We had conversations.

James loved conversations, he told me. His house had been a noisy one, full of voices and clamouring, and as the youngest he had never been given a chance to speak. It was chaotic, which he loved, but he'd longed for silence.

I thought that was funny, it was like the inverse of my house, where the silence was oppressive, I'd longed for noise.

Falling in love with James had a rhythm; it was as though we'd always been existing on the same plane, like we were reflections of each other.

When I returned from London, we both knew that our future was to be together. James asked if I would move to London, but I told him that I couldn't move for someone again. He was disappointed, but he said he understood. 'I just need more time,' I said.

This was Hong Kong all over again, one of my friends warned me. I also saw the patterns. Like Drew, James represented possibility, he lived across an ocean, he was asking me to move for him. But why was I so convinced that James was different? How did I know?

It went beyond James being different from Drew. I understood that for James, there was truth. He was clear-sighted, a true scientist, and just as my mother had known that with my father his love for her would be clear, I knew that with James everything would be logical and proven. James saw life as something to build, to create. And I knew that a life with him would be one which we would create together, without any predetermined rules.

James loved to live in the moment. 'Let's take in this moment,' he'd say, and we'd breathe in, taking in the sounds, the smells, the stillness in the air. He helped me capture time.

I felt so happy with James, I couldn't help but wonder what the cost would be. What would the fates decide would be the price of feeling pure joy. My grandmother's warning was in my ear, but I pushed away the feeling and the doubt, I decided to believe.

I met James' family at Christmas time. Their house in New Jersey was decorated with tinsel and plastic lights. James' mother was tall like him, lean, with a continual moving energy, her normal state was one of perpetual motion. She was a homemaker who was devoted to her three sons. James was the youngest, the baby of the family, and her unquestioned favourite. He was the only one who had her love of adventure, she said.

James' father was a paediatrician with a private practice in New York. He was jolly, with a booming laugh and a constant smile. He was a devout Christian. He loved to show us Pinterest quotes about faith, and he had Bible verses painted on the walls of the house.

I was initially nervous to meet them. I knew the rules of a Korean daughter-in-law, I was meant to be subservient and obedient, quiet and never questioning of authority. It was obvious that they knew the rules too, but I soon learned that I wasn't expected to play the game. They were welcoming, warm and excited to meet the girl that James had brought home. James had told them we had fallen in love at first conversation, but they didn't seem concerned about the speed of our meeting. Perhaps it was because they had married a week after they'd met; it was an arranged marriage.

We spoke in English, which eliminated the need for the formal tense in Korean, and they treated me as a friend rather than a daughter-in-law that they could scold.

'What are the qualities you look for most in a man?' James' father asked me.

I thought for a moment; I thought of Drew, and I thought of James. What was it that I saw in James?

'I would like three things,' I said. 'Kindness, loyalty and conviction.'

He laughed heartily. 'Conviction? James has a lot of conviction. That can make life difficult.' He looked thoughtful. 'But he has kindness.'

I would meet the rest of James' family over the Christmas period, a loud raucous clan. It was exhilarating – cousins, aunts, uncles all in one house in New Jersey. We played card games and drank beer. There were always tables of food, we'd eat with Styrofoam plates on our laps. Children would run screaming through the rooms, and the grown-ups would shout and laugh.

One afternoon, James asked me to walk outside with him. 'I need a moment,' he said. 'It's too much.' We put on our coats and walked in the cold air, trudging along the snowbanks, looking at the houses draped in Christmas lights.

I took James to my home to meet my parents, we took the train down to Washington DC. It was like entering a different world. My parents' house was monastic, quiet, the silence echoed off the wooden floors. My father asked James to step closer so that he could see him. 'I can't see well,' he explained, and he took off his glasses and looked at James hard.

James didn't seem nervous; he talked with my father about mathematics and the piano. My father seemed relieved, in his element, while my mother chatted excitedly with me over tea.

At one point, I said to James, 'It's so quiet, it must be strange.'

'No, I like it,' James said. 'I can think.'

And we greeted the New Year in silence. No television or ball drop, just the distant sound of fireworks in the background.

After quitting my job and starting freelance work, I decided to move to New York. I moved into a small living room in Queens, where I slept on the floor in a sleeping bag. New York was sprawling, anonymous but familiar, always an open city for whoever seeks refuge.

I met up with James' mother often in the city. It began as a whim; she called me to ask if I wanted to get coffee. She took me to a cafe in Little Italy, where we wandered the alleyways until we found the place she swore had the best pastries. We had espressos and shared cannoli. Spending time with her reminded me of James. She told me that she loved to take the bus into New York and wander the neighbourhoods on her own. She would choose a new neighbourhood to explore, and she'd enter every single shop, walk down the back streets and get lost. 'James would follow me when he was little,' she said. 'He loved to walk with me.' She sounded wistful.

We started to meet often in the city. She took me to the coffee shops she loved in the Bronx, where we'd share hot buns and empanadas. We sat in a booth and listened to the chatter of Spanish.

'It reminds me of Argentina,' she said. 'It's where I grew up.' I learned that she had left Korea when she was thirteen. Her mother was the one who'd decided that she would have an arranged marriage. Her mother had chosen James' father because he was a doctor and a Christian, elements of a good husband.

'I feel lucky to be with him,' she said. 'He's a good man.' She smiled at me.

We did have our occasional misunderstandings. James' mother had a habit of making comments and criticisms that would stay under my skin. 'Why are you wearing this?' she asked me once, when I came to a family birthday party wearing flats. 'We need to go shopping so that you can make a good impression.' I found out later that she was concerned that I hadn't made a good impression on her mother-in-law, James' grandmother.

Why didn't I care more about what people thought? Her comments and implications frustrated me. I had thought I didn't have to contend with the rules, but I could feel the burden of tradition, the borders coming down, and the generations of expectation weighing on me.

But the comment that bothered me the most was that I needed to learn to 'surrender'.

'When you're married, you have to adapt,' she'd warn me. 'You have to surrender.'

'I surrender' was her most common phrase. She'd say it and laugh when she talked about her husband or her sons. Why? I'd think. Why surrender? And I'd think to myself, I'd refuse, no matter what.

I didn't mention my annoyance to my mother, because I knew what she would say. She would just be angry and tell me that she'd warned me about mothers-in-law, and she'd tell me the Korean stories about their cruelty. 'In-laws,' she'd say, and her eyes would flash darkly.

I remembered her story about my father's family. On a visit after her marriage, she'd gone alone to their house to help prepare for my grandfather's sixtieth birthday. They took her passport and kept her in their house against her will, intending to train her to be a good wife and daughter-in-law. When they finally let her return to the US, she had to be hospitalised – whether for exhaustion or stress, I'm not sure. My father refused to speak to them for years.

So whenever James' mother talked about surrendering, I'd think of the Korean folk tales, I'd think of my mother and her stories. But then James' mother and I would laugh again over coffee, and I'd wonder if I'd only imagined the tension.

Meanwhile, James and I took turns visiting one another. I washed dishes at parties, tutored and freelanced to save money for my flights. Each time I visited London it would feel like no time had passed at all, there had been a parallel existence waiting for me. It was a strange feeling, I no longer knew where home was. Each time I stepped inside the airport, it was like stepping through a doorway.

James proposed later that year. It was spring, and the trees were tipped with frost. He gave me a journal he'd been keeping for months about our relationship, and a ring that shone like a star.

When James asked my mother if he should ask my father for permission to marry me, she told him not to bother. 'It's Catherine's decision.'

We called Teddy to tell him the news. He was hiking in Nepal. 'Cool,' he said. His voice sounded wistful over the phone.

My mother seemed happy for me, for us. Neither of my parents commented that James was a professor like my father, and if they saw any similarities in our stories, they kept it quiet. My mother never asked me why it didn't work out in Hong Kong, she seemed to accept that it was a closed door.

James and I were married exactly a year from the day we met, at City Hall in San Francisco. We chose San Francisco by chance because it was the location of another friend's wedding. James flew in from London, and I flew in from New York. We went to the friend's wedding, where we danced to jazz and cheered for the slow-motion camera booth. The next day, dressed in the outfits we'd been wearing on the night we met, we took a taxi to City Hall. James looked nervous in his tux and groomsman tie, and I was wearing a black and white dress. I was holding hydrangeas that I'd taken from the centrepieces at our friend's wedding; they were a shade of pale blue. It was just the two of us and two friends as witnesses. I felt nervous and shaky, I tried breathing, slow counts.

As we climbed the stairs of City Hall, I remembered the moment we'd met. I thought of us as children, James the youngest of three brothers longing for silence, me chasing fireflies with Teddy. My life with James felt steady and safe and certain. There had been no sorrow, no need for sacrifice. I wondered what my grandmother would think if she could see us, holding hands as we climbed the marble steps.

We stood across from one another, like reflections. The judge spoke a few words, and we were married.

I gave my hydrangeas to a couple we met on the way outside. 'It can be your something borrowed and blue!' I said. 'Pass it on!' James and I beamed at each other; we were giddy. We toasted our marriage with pancakes and champagne at a nearby diner, and then we headed to the airport, and I flew back to New York and James to London.

I would move to London a few months later, strangely enough on a New Year's Eve. This time instead of crossing the Pacific, I was crossing the Atlantic. And instead of Drew, it was James. A mirror. On the plane, there was no countdown to midnight; it was as though we were suspended above time again. And I knew that when I landed it'd be morning, a beginning.

I moved into James' small studio with two suitcases of belongings. I spent my days walking through Hyde Park and the halls of the Victoria and Albert Museum. I looked at the gathered items and wondered at these objects, so fragile, that had somehow been preserved through time. A collection of hand mirrors, a pen, a piece of cloth. If my life were a collection of objects, I didn't know what they would be. I felt like I'd been untethered, but was now linked to the world through James. I knew he wouldn't let me go.

At our London wedding for our family and friends a year later, our first dance was a swing dance to Ray Charles. James wore braces, and I twirled around the dance floor in trainers. We served bourbon in cut glasses, the night shone like a jewel.

It wasn't a fairy tale; I still had nightmares. Nightmares so vivid that I'd wake up covered in sweat as though I'd been running. I'd wake up convinced I was still in Hong Kong, that I was still with Drew, and I'd scream and shout as I thought I was being suffocated. James was patient; he'd listen to me, and he'd remind me gently of our life together; we'd talk until I was no longer afraid.

It's evening. I can tell because it's medication time.

I stand in line and obediently swallow the bitter liquid, knowing to chase it with a cup of Sunny Delight this time. My eyes are heavy, and my mouth is dry.

I wait to see if James will call again, but when I lift the receiver there's no dial tone.

Someone comes in and shuts off the lights in the TV room, and one by one we shuffle out. The worker in front of my room makes a note on her clipboard, and she nods at me as she closes the door.

Even though I know it isn't, it feels like my first night in the ward. I feel aware of the sounds, the silences, the sheets. I stand silently by the bed, unsure if I should undress. A part of me moves mechanically as I brush my teeth, jamming my toothbrush in the divot by the sink to make the water run. The fluorescent lighting is harsh against my skin, and I express milk into the sink quickly with shaking hands.

I keep my clothing on, the sweater feels reassuring, familiar. The sheets scratch against my cheek, and I feel a sudden ache for home, my own bed.

There's a sliver of light from the outside hallway. I can hear slamming doors, someone is screaming, there are muffled shouts. My door opens, and I close my eyes and lie still and tensed. The door closes again, and I let out my breath as I realise it was probably a worker doing a headcount.

I am weary, my body is heavy, and I can feel my eyes closing. I try to think of home, I try to think of before, how I got here, but it feels raw, an exposed tangle of thoughts.

What would I be doing if I wasn't here? I think of Cato, I have a glimpse of him in my mind. And I have a memory, a feeling, an imprint of holding a baby in my arms. I try to picture his face, but my body folds with an ache so hard it is like a part of me is hollow. I retreat from it and am thankful for the dark.

I decide to pay more attention to my surroundings.

The workers' faces are blurred. I learn them first by their hairstyles and then eventually their faces as they come in focus. Most of the workers are immigrants, from the Caribbean and Africa. They speak English with a hard lilt. Sometimes they laugh with one another and speak in their own languages.

There's Jean, with a blunt bob and straight bangs. She is tough with a 'take no bullshit' attitude. She speaks with a snap in her tone, but she's also one of the most generous on the ward. She buys treats for us with her own money, bringing them out in the cafeteria with a stern look and a pretend reluctance. Her attitude and sympathy for us make me wonder if she grew up in the system.

There's Nona, with thin, wavy dark hair and a voice like a bird's. She was the one to first take me to the shower room, stripping my clothes off and chattering to me in broken English. 'No, no,' she shouted at me when I tried to turn the tap for the water. She handed me a toothbrush which I jammed into a divot in the side of the shower tap in order to turn on the water. It was icy.

'Breasts, breasts,' she shouted, gesturing at me to press them. I did so gingerly, the knots were deep and swollen.

'You have to get better so you can go home to baby,' she said.

None of them seem fazed by us, and I know the other residents respect that about them. The only exception is

Claire, a young blonde nurse who is on rotation. She is nervous around us; we can smell it. She doesn't look us in the eye and is careful not to let us brush past her. She often says the wrong thing. 'Tamyra? You're here again? I feel like every time I'm here, you're here too!' She says it playfully and then falters.

Mick stifles a smirk, and Tamyra glares and then smiles falsely, too brightly. She starts to follow Claire around, stands as close as possible to her without touching. She sniffs Claire's neck, Claire freezes, she acts like you would when faced with a rabid dog.

Every morning, Claire takes our blood pressure and our heart rate. She sets up a chair in front of the glass enclosure and calls us over one by one, checking our names off a clipboard. I sit on the chair, and she fusses around me quickly, like she doesn't want to do the wrong thing. I want to tell her to relax and I smile at her, but she's carefully looking away from me, like I'm contagious.

We are walking to lunch. Jenny is sitting on the floor, crying in the hallway. She's shivering so hard her mouth is moving. Jenny came in this morning. She's a pretty mother of two, in her early thirties, with dark, teased hair and smudged eyeliner. She has two front teeth, but the rest are brown and rotted.

When she came in this morning, she glanced around the room and then came over to speak to Emma and me. Jenny is white, and she has a job at Target. She uses this to hold herself apart from the others. I think she knows Tamyra, they nodded at each other, but kept their distance.

I wonder about all the residents in the ward. What would it be like if we'd met outside? I know they think of me as someone who doesn't belong, not with my advanced degree, my brand-name leggings. I have a home. I have someone waiting for me. I'm privileged. Even Jenny, with her rotted teeth and shaking hands, she's privileged.

Sometimes the others look at me in a way that makes me feel guilty. I'm lucky, I know it.

'I see you,' Ali had said to me again this morning. 'I see what you're doing. You're being smart.'

I don't ask what he means, because I know. He's doing the same thing.

We don't belong. We keep our heads down.

I think of this as I see Jenny shivering on the floor.

'You OK?' Will asks.

Jenny shakes her head while shivering. 'They won't give me my meds,' she says.

When we come back out of the cafeteria, the paramedics are here. We see Jenny on the floor. 'Step back,' one of the workers says.

'What's happened?' Emma asks. She's sliding in her socks.

'I think she's had a seizure,' Will says quietly.

'Step back,' the worker repeats. The paramedics are standing over Jenny, blocking our view. They act like they can't see us watching.

Dessert today is sliced canned pineapple.

My mother used to tell me that when my grandfather was drunk he would go buy cans of pineapple. It was a luxury, and my grandmother would scold him and cry, how would she feed the children this week? But my mother would clap her hands – pineapple!

When I was sick, my mother would crush Tylenol in orange juice to cut the bitterness and give me slices of pineapple circles in a crystal dish.

She would never have any though.

Tamyra doesn't want mine, and so I eat it as slowly as I dare, savouring the sweetness on my tongue.

Darren joins me at the activity table. His eyes keep darting around the room and his hands are shaking. There is a Chinese Checkers board on the table. 'Ma'am, you know how to play?' he asks.

I nod. 'Do you want me to teach you?' I ask.

He smiles, and for a moment his handsome face looks like a child's. Emma still avoids him, ever since he lunged at her, and I notice that the others keep their distance. I don't know if it's gang-related, but then I wonder if I'm being prejudiced by automatically assuming he's in a gang. One of the Hispanic patients referred to Darren as 'Trayvon', which I recognise as a reference to his dark hoodie. Behind Darren's smile I can glimpse a volatile light, as though there's something just out of reach, waiting to be uncaged. He is shy around me, as if I'm fragile, and he speaks to me like I'm a headmistress.

The Chinese Checkers pieces are neon colours, too bright, and both of us shade our eyes from the board.

I can't remember the rules, and so I teach the game wrong, I can't remember if you can jump forwards or backwards, but we move the pieces along the board, and Darren laughs whenever he jumps one of mine.

There is a moment when he looks upset that I jumped one of his pieces, and he seems tensed, a muscle in his jaw twitches, but then he looks at me and sticks out his tongue playfully and relaxes.

'He your brother?' he asks me.

'My brother?'

He nods and points at Haru, who is colouring in a unicorn. Haru looks half Asian, I'm not sure how long he's been on the ward, but he acts as though he lives here. He is sweet and deliberate, but he can throw a tantrum when it's time for *Criminal Intent* – that's his show and he never misses it.

Haru looks confused. 'You thought I was her brother?' He looks at me. 'Am I?'

'No,' I say. 'No, Haru, we aren't related.'

Ali's family comes in to the ward. They have weary eyes, and they sit at the conference table in the activity room with Christine, the social worker. Ali paces and then stands by the glass. I can see that Ali looks like his father, tall and lean. His father has an arm around Ali's mother, who wears a veil and keeps her eyes on the ground. Neither of them glance in his direction, it's like he doesn't exist.

'Is that your family?' Mick asks. He's wheeled his wheelchair up to the glass.

'Yeah.'

'Are they OK?'

'No, they're worried, man, they're worried.'

Mick nods. Ali looks like a child, waiting for someone to nod and say hello. His parents leave without looking at him. I look for him later, but he's lying in his room. When he comes out for dinner, his eyes are red and swollen.

I learn from group that not everyone has family who are waiting for them or helping them to get out. That is a rarity. There is Mick, whose brother is helping him but who doesn't want to be saddled with him once he's out. 'Don't blame him,' Mick says gruffly. Tamyra's boyfriend is watching her kids. He calls her once a day, but she doesn't always answer the phone. 'Tell him I'm busy,' she says and rolls her eyes. Emma's father calls her every few hours while the phone is on, I'm guessing he also has an 'avocado'.

We don't talk about how we're going to leave. That would mean acknowledging that there is a world outside. But I know everyone is thinking about it. They must be, I think. I can sense that the question of how to leave is not something I can ask. The returners seem to know, but they don't share the information with us, and they watch silently as Emma flips through her papers and shows me a new form that she's filled in.

Emma is the only one who talks about leaving, her strategy, her countdown. 'I'm going to move up to level two,' she says. 'I just need someone to sign this, it says that I've made a new friend. I have to get three signatures. Will you sign it?'

'My avocado is going to get us all out of here,' she says. 'All of us.'

The only one who seems to believe her is Dave. He trails her in his wheelchair. The others ignore her.

We act like we are meant to be here, like we've just happened to appear. We are existing in this place, with nowhere else to go.

I stare at the doctors and workers standing behind the glass, but they are careful not to meet my eyes, and when they look up, they look through me as though I am transparent. I give up after trying to linger by the glass enclosure. I imagine myself shouting at them: 'Let me out, let me out.' I know that would just be a ticket to stay.

I am colouring a lion in purple Crayola marker. Next to me, Emma is filing through her papers yet again, trying to stick tabs on them – an impossible task as she's using tissues.

'Catherine,' Jeff says. 'Your husband is here.' I hear Tamyra hiss. I look around me, but no one else stands up for visiting hour.

I walk through the hallway, counting my steps – there are fifty-four – one foot after the other towards the cafeteria door.

For a moment, I'm afraid of who I will see, will it be Drew? But it's James' anxious face in the window of the cafeteria door. He looks haggard, but he's beaming.

'Are we allowed to touch?' I ask.

'Yes.' Jeff nods.

James embraces me. It's like he's brought in air from the outside, oxygen.

I take a deep breath in and try to ground myself in James, in the certainty that is him. I can feel the past and present. It feels secure, a foundation, and I want to disappear in his arms.

I hear murmurs, I see Emma and Mick, they also have visitors, but all I can do is focus on James.

James isn't speaking; he's just holding my hand.

We sit, and I'm just breathing in this moment.

'Thank you for the sweaters,' I say. 'What are you wearing?' I ask. 'Do you have enough clothes?'

'Stop it,' he says. 'Stop worrying about me. Did you get the notebook?'

'Yes,' I say.

He tells me that he's been calling the ward every day, many times a day, working on getting me out, asking about my status.

'I've been making myself a pain in the ass,' he says.

I laugh, because I know that he's been approaching this the way he would one of his research projects. He was the one to think of leaving me a notebook, which he had to lobby for, and he argued for them to give me a pen. He dropped off my glasses when he realised I didn't have them with me.

'I've been handling the insurance,' he says hesitantly. 'So don't worry about that.' He tells me that he's been on the phone to the UK, to my GP to get my paperwork released, he's been on the phone with the travel insurance companies, trying to log in to my computer and credit cards with my combination of passwords. His words make me think of the outside world, how it's continuing on, all the logistics and mechanisms, somehow it keeps going.

'Don't you want to know about Cato?' he asks.

'Yes, how's Cato?' I'd forgotten. The name doesn't have significance to me.

'He's good, he's good. They wouldn't let me bring a phone in, but I printed some photos of him for you.' He hands me a stack of photos. I glance at them; I see a chubby-faced baby with wide eyes. I don't recognise him. I tuck the photos in the pocket of my hoodie.

'I spoke to the nurses, you can keep them with you,' James says. 'I told them it'd help you.'

He pauses. 'Do you remember what happened? We don't have to talk about it now,' he says quickly.

'I remember a lot,' I say. 'But it's confusing.'

He waits.

'I drew a family tree,' I offer.

He starts to cry. I feel a twinge of something, but I don't know what to do, so I just pat his hand.

'It's just that … we kept trying to get you to draw one, but you couldn't.'

Visiting hour is over. It feels like we've just sat down. 'Time's up,' Jeff says it gruffly, but his eyes are soft. 'Let's wrap things up, guys.'

James sighs.

He holds my hand until the last moment. He smiles widely, but I can see that he's still crying. 'I'll see you soon, I promise.' He walks towards the doors while waving to me, and he's still looking at me waving to him when they close.

It occurs to me that I didn't ask him how long I'd have to stay.

They shuffle us out of the room, back to the ward, back to the waiting place.

There is one Korean fairy tale about romantic love. Jiknyeo, a sky-maiden, falls in love with a herder, Gyeonwu. She glimpses him from across the Milky Way. She begs her father, the sky-king, to let them be married. Her father agrees.

The lovers are married. They are so happy and in love that they neglect their duties. In anger and to punish them, the sky-king orders them to live apart. But he shows one act of mercy: on the seventh day of the seventh month of each year they will be allowed to meet.

When the seventh day of the seventh month arrives, the lovers are desperate to see one another, but they cannot cross the Milky Way. A flock of magpies form a bridge for the lovers to meet.

And so each year, for one night, the lovers are reunited. This night marks the start of the rainy season; if it rains on that night, it is meant to be the couple's tears.

I found out I was pregnant on a grey day in February. My period was late, but I was convinced it was a fluke. I decided to take a pregnancy test, thinking that once I'd spent money on the test, my period would come with a vengeance. Instead, it read positive. It was a Tuesday morning and my husband was straightening his shirt, headed to a work meeting.

I wasn't sure how to feel. I was thirty years old, the same age as my mother when she had me, and the same age as my grandmother when she had my mother. It felt preordained. The idea of being a mother had always felt vague to me, I knew it was something I wanted, but I'd never thought deeply about it. It was an idea, something I'd had to imagine and now it was real.

I made an appointment with the GP. It was five weeks, the baby was a mass of cells, the size of a poppy seed.

When we told our parents, my mother was in disbelief. 'Really?' she said. My father didn't comment. James' parents screamed and clapped. 'How wonderful,' they said. 'How wonderful.'

I started counting time in weeks. Each week was a new fruit, I watched my body swell from poppy seed to watermelon.

We went to the appointments, the ultrasound scans. I tested positive for gestational diabetes, and so several times a day I had to prick my finger on a paper strip and count my blood sugar levels. Each time I collected a drop of blood, I thought of Snow White, and I wondered what I should wish for for my child.

When I found out I was having a boy, I thought of Drew. Actually, I thought of Leah, and for the first time, instead of anger, I felt sympathy. How would it feel, to have something of my own creation, a beautiful thing, become twisted and dirty and abusive?

The poisoned part of me, the part I'd taken from Drew, was it still there? Would it infect the baby? I'd read that an ancestor's experience is imprinted in the DNA of the next generation, a warning for what was to come. Was violence there? Was an acceptance of suffering? Would my son be afraid of heights? Would he have nightmares of suffocating? How were we meant to exit the loops of the past if we were destined to face them again and again?

I thought of my family, my own ancestors. They were a mystery to me, one that I didn't know about, separated by language and ocean, I only knew them in my own features. I wondered what my grandmother felt when she was pregnant with my mother – the fear, the hope for a son.

For some reason, I'd thought that I'd be having a girl, a third-generation daughter to pass on the stories, but perhaps this boy was an answer to my grandmother's wish, imprinted on generations. I held my hands close to my stomach and tried to feel the tiny beats of his legs, the pulse of his body, the reminder that he was alive, a living thing.

James played music to my stomach; he'd read a study that music heard during pregnancy could calm the baby outside of the womb. We learned that Rachmaninoff made him jump and that he would do flips to Broadway musicals. It was strange to watch my skin ripple with each tug, a being doing somersaults inside.

Pregnancy felt like a separation from the body. My body was doing something on its own, a pre-programmed path it already knew, and I no longer had any control over. It felt like a hand sharply bringing my spirit back to my body, a return to the earthiness of it. It was also an erasure of self; I didn't feel more 'me', I felt like I was being split, being shared. My body was no longer my own, I was a carrier, a holder of life. It was a reminder that my body was a collection of blood and bones.

'I like cervixes,' a smiling midwife said to me while her hand was still inside me performing my fourth membrane sweep.

I was induced two days before my due date. It was a decision made by doctors because of my gestational diabetes and the concern that the baby was measuring big.

'We would have to break the shoulders,' a doctor said to me helpfully. I learned that doctors had a way of saying horrific things matter-of-factly. I agreed to the induction.

We checked into the hospital like we were checking into a hotel. We had luggage, a car seat for the baby and a stack of books and magazines. We sat in the hospital room and listened to the hum of the lights and beeping of monitors. I was taken to a bed in a ward with four other women. We were all waiting for our inductions. I was hooked up to machines to monitor my blood pressure and heart rate. The induction started with a pessary containing prostaglandin, a hormone that is meant to trigger labour. A midwife inserted the cotton wool in me, and I lay in the bed and wondered how it would feel to give birth. I could hear the shifting of women's bodies and the sounds of their monitors. Every few hours a nurse would arrive to take my temperature and check my heart rate.

I started having contractions quickly, I watched the waves on the monitors, the small swells that corresponded to the tightening of a fist around my body. 'You have a high pain tolerance,' one of the midwives said to me cheerfully. 'Look!' She pointed at a wave that was reaching a high peak. 'Maybe you should walk around, it will help encourage labour.'

I learned that the success of an induction is measured by the shortest route to labour. If the pessary didn't work, then I would have to have another pessary inserted after twelve hours. The induction process would keep escalating until a baby was born.

James and I left the ward to walk the hallways, pacing back and forth along the corridor that loomed over us. There was no outside light, only the bright fluorescence of the hospital lights. It felt like an empty chamber. I walked, and every few steps I'd have to stop as a contraction took over.

'Only two centimetres,' a midwife said after checking how far I was dilated. 'Can I give you another sweep?' I agreed and tried to relax as she moved her hand inside me. I was a body, I was strong, I could do this. Another pessary was inserted, and again I paced the hallways.

We played a game of questions.

'What qualities do you want him to have?' James asked. 'I think you would say strength and kindness.'

'Yes, you're right.' With strength and kindness, one could face the world. We had already chosen his name, James had chosen Cato for the Roman statesman, and I had chosen his middle name, Westbrook, for my godfather, a World War II veteran and linguistics professor. Strength and kindness.

We paced slowly, while I stopped every few breaths to lean over and count until the waves subsided.

I counted my steps, and I thought of those thousand steps in Hong Kong. What had I thought would happen if I'd been able to cross them?

I thought of Jiknyeo walking over the magpies across the Milky Way to meet her love. Just one more step, I'd think. Just another, that's all that was separating me from becoming a mother. I still didn't know how it would feel. I couldn't imagine it.

By the morning, I was dilated enough to start labour. We carried our luggage to another floor, while I chatted with a midwife who talked about labour like it was a party.

'We'll need to break your waters,' she said. 'It may be uncomfortable.' I could tell from her voice that she was lying.

She broke my waters with a long hook the size of an umbrella. I managed not to flinch.

She hooked me up to more machines and a hormone drip to encourage more contractions. There was a clock on the wall, and I tried to count the hours, punctuated by the buzzing of the monitors and the waves of my contractions.

I had an hour of strong contractions, ones that I tried to ride like waves. My husband held my hands as I breathed, in and out, and waited for the epidural. The epidural was a cold thread in my spine, my legs and feet were numb, but I could still feel them. The contractions felt like faint echoes, I could no longer feel the pain.

The hours kept passing, my cervix had been checked so many times I no longer dreaded it.

My temperature and heart rate started to climb dangerously, and I developed sepsis. The midwife sat next to me, trying to hide the concern on her face as she counted the heartbeats.

A doctor came and introduced herself.

Why am I meeting a doctor? I thought.

'It's just in case we need to work together tonight.'

She introduced her whole team: an anaesthesiologist, two junior doctors, a paediatric nurse.

'We'll be back,' she said.

I had a feeling that they knew that I would need a C-section.

There was another hour, and the doctor returned to check my cervix again.

'You're only four centimetres dilated,' she said, 'and it looks like it's not progressing. I think that the best way forward might be a C-section. What do you think?'

I noticed that her arm was dripping in blood. I agreed.

'Good,' she said, and before I realised what was happening, her team rushed into the room and moved me on to a gurney. 'One, two, three.'

Next to me, James had put on scrubs.

Finally, we thought, finally this was going to happen.

Time seemed to flip forward, the team was sprinting with the stretcher, pushing me into an operating theatre.

'You're going to feel cold,' the anaesthesiologist said. 'Do you have any loose teeth?'

I shook my head.

'OK,' the anaesthesiologist said. She sprayed a bottle on me. 'Do you feel anything?'

'No,' I said.

I started shaking and chattering uncontrollably. The anaesthesiologist spoke calmly in my ear.

'Your stomach will feel like someone is looking for something in a handbag,' she said.

I remember the moment of seeing our son, he was red and squalling, and I remember thinking vaguely, are you sure? He didn't look like either of us. There were some concerns with his breathing, and James was running back and forth between me and the baby. I was dry heaving, trying to vomit into a bucket, still shaking uncontrollably.

They took the baby to check his breathing, and I was wheeled to a recovery ward. I hadn't eaten since the night before, and I ordered a sandwich. There wasn't a bed for James, so he slept by me again in a chair.

I'd said to James before, isn't it funny how everyone says mother and baby are happy and healthy?

'What should we say?' he asked the next morning.

'Just say that mother and baby are happy and healthy,' I said. I understood why everyone said that, it was simpler.

After a mother gives birth in Korea, she is immediately rushed to her bed, covered with blankets and kept warm. She is given seaweed soup made with a strong beef-bone broth. The seaweed is meant to give her strength. It is your mother who is meant to make you this soup, she will wash the seaweed again and again to wash away the grit of the ocean.

Every year on your birthday, you drink this soup in honour of your mother's suffering. It is 'mother's soup'.

I remember that on my birthday, my mother would make seaweed soup for me. She would soak the strands of dried seaweed, carefully picked from a Korean supermarket. I'd watch her boil the beef stock as she washed the seaweed again and again. And when I tasted it, I felt like I could taste the ocean.

I was also born by C-section. My mother told me I was clinging to her; I was born over a month late. The doctor cut my mother vertically, the way you would slice a melon. Growing up, I'd thought the scar was beautiful, it reminded me of a braid woven along her body.

My scar is horizontal, the length of a hand along my hipbone. It heals and fades to a raised pink line, the colour of a shell.

When the midwives brought Cato to me, he was red-faced with a full head of dark hair. He looked at me with alert, round eyes as though he knew who I was already.

I didn't feel a rush of love or an overwhelming weight of responsibility, emotions that I'd been expecting. Instead, I felt curious, like I'd just been introduced to a stranger. He was a creature, an idea, not even human yet, just a being, a life.

The nurse helped unfasten my hospital robe and put him on my chest.

I felt a rush of living, of being alive in the moment. Suspended.

My stomach was the shape of a square, the doctors had pressed on the uterus to tighten it.

Around me, I heard women crying and the faint sounds of mewling babies.

'Hold him for a while,' the nurse said.

And I held him, close.

I could feel his breath against my skin, his tiny hands were clutching for me, as though he knew that we'd been cut apart. I hummed to him, hoping the vibrations would soothe him. James was standing next to me, taking deep breaths, his hand on my shoulder. Cato was so small, he felt so fragile in my arms, like he didn't belong in this world. His hair was dark, the colour of night, so dark it had glints of silver and red, and he looked up at me with his eyes unblinking. His eyes had a depth, a dimension beyond oceans. He looked at me without any expression, I looked back at him in wonder.

I thought we'd be going home soon, but we had to stay for another week in the hospital so that Cato could finish a course of antibiotics. The doctors were worried that he had developed an infection from my sepsis. They were taking precautions.

The labour ward was a bright room of eight beds separated by plastic curtains. It was a cacophony of mothers and babies. Each day the doctors came by with clipboards and told me that I could leave, and each day I'd pack up our things only for them to extend our stay.

I had a catheter, but no one had told me that it needed to be removed straight away, and someone had forgotten to remove mine. I ended up buzzing for a nurse to change the bag of urine. 'You still have the catheter in?' she asked. 'It needs to be taken out now!' I spent the next day trying to pass urine, feeling panicked because it wasn't happening, and sure that my bladder was going to explode.

I was so constantly being groped and poked and told to do skin-to-skin that eventually I just took off my clothes and sat on the bed with the baby on my chest. I felt mammalian; there to exist, just to do what I'd been told.

My scar burned, I could feel it, a broad slash across my abdomen. I could feel the metal wiring stitching it together, sometimes I wanted to touch it, the way we want to examine an open wound, but I refrained. It hurt to sit up, and each time Cato leaned on me, my stomach would form into a different shape, developing sharp corners.

I'd thought I would reclaim my body after birth, but instead, it was now a tool, something to sustain life. My physical self was just to give, to provide sustenance for this new being. It was more than draining. My body, my mind, everything was focused on Cato. In the blur of those hours, I stopped thinking of myself as having a name, I was a body. I had no identity, I was just a number on the marker board and a set of vitals. A nurse came every hour to take my blood pressure and heart rate, which she'd mark wordlessly on a chart, sweeping the curtains behind her as she left. It felt like every few moments those curtains were being opened, and a new face would arrive and ask me what I was doing and how I was doing it.

Next to me, through the curtains, I could hear some of the women crying. 'I'm not an animal,' one of them said.

'Why aren't you listening to me?' another said.

I was sympathetic. Our identities had been overwritten. Each of us had brought a new life into the world, but we were all the same in this shared experience.

I rarely saw the other mothers, they were just voices to me. I knew them by their moaning, by the sound of their quiet cries. Sometimes we'd pass each other in the halls, taking small, steps painful in our paper slippers, and we'd nod to each other, knowing that we were bleeding. We were in this place, waiting to leave. It was another suspended place, and we were here, just existing.

Time was marked by feeding and not feeding, punctuated by medication times, which I could tell were approaching when the sharp aches in my body became almost unbearable. I could hear the rattle of the medication cart, and the midwife who measured out the pills in small plastic cups. I could hear the woman in the bed next to mine sobbing while waiting for it to arrive.

'You can go to her first,' I said.

The midwife looked at me and shook her head. 'Everyone has their turn.'

The days passed in rotation: feeding, not feeding. I lost track of the days and nights, it was just a continuous blur. Cato would scream and scream in hunger, insistent, primal. Feeding was relentless, it would take an hour of wrestling just to get Cato to latch on, and then the moment he stopped, it'd only be time for him to be fed again. My body ached, my scar was a searing brand on my body, and my breasts were swollen and raw.

I wore compression socks, tightly wrapped around my legs. My feet swelled up as though filled with water.

I didn't leave the ward, but James came in and out from the outside. He brought back trays of sushi and cold beer. We made a toast to the baby, our own private celebration.

At night, the lights were kept on, and I could hear the sound of the machines and the faint whir of the lights. I grew used to the sound of the curtains opening and the footsteps of the nurses who came in to do their checks, and the sound of babies crying, which was constant.

It was cold, the heater was broken and the vents were pouring out freezing air.

Cato was in a small plastic cot next to me. I'd lie on my side and stare at him, wrapped in his hat and swaddled in a blanket. He had his fists tucked under his chin, escaping from the swaddle, as though he was in a boxing stance, ready to take on the world. He wasn't sleeping; he shivered in his hat and looked at me with his round eyes.

'We're in this together,' I said to him. I felt like we were prisoners, but we will escape the ward, I said. I'd reach a hand over to him, but the cot was too far away, and I knew that getting out of bed would hurt. So instead, I'd watch him struggle in his swaddle, crying and crying, insistent and desperate, and after a while I'd manoeuvre myself out of the bed and gasp in pain when I bent over to lift him. I'd turn the lever of the bed to be upright, so that I could sit up with Cato in my arms. I'd pinch myself to stay awake, and I'd whisper stories to Cato while he slept. I'd tell him the Western fairy tales, the ones I loved best, but then I'd find myself telling him the stories my mother and my grandmother used to tell me. I told him about the rabbit who tricked the king who wanted to eat his liver. The woodcutter who trapped a sky-maiden, only to have her leave with their children, taken back to the sky in a stream of ribbons. I told him the stories of sacrifice, of a love so true that it could only cause pain.

I wondered how my grandmother had told my mother these stories. Could she have guessed that they would be told again? Except this time in another language, crossing two oceans, to an old world. As I looked at Cato in my arms, all the hope we had in this one life, I thought of Drew's mother. At one time he must have seemed like this, uncorrupted, pure. She must have whispered stories to him and promised him her love. She must have dreamed of his future; she must have seen oceans in his eyes.

Sometimes, if Cato wouldn't sleep, I'd put on my paper slippers and wander the halls with him wrapped in a blanket. I'd hold him close to me, pacing the lighted corridors. We could hear the buzzing of the lights, the murmurs of babies and nurses. As we walked, I could feel my heart beating against his body, and I wondered whether he was starting to feel alone, his world was just expanding, with each step there was more to see, more to discover, more to fear.

We were released just as night fell on a Friday. It was a little over a week since I'd checked in to the hospital. I felt triumphant; it was exhilarating to finally leave the ward. I stood on the street and listened to the rush of cars, to the sound of the city. I wanted to scream in the pure exhilaration of it. James hugged me, he was holding Cato, and we looked at each other in dismay. They were letting us leave with this human creature, what were we meant to do now?

We sat in the cab, Cato buckled into the car seat.

'Congratulations,' our cabbie said. He promised to go slowly, and he grinned, excited to be driving a newborn. 'So, Mum, how does it feel?' I didn't have a clear answer, I stared into the city night. The lights felt sharper, the air felt clearer, it was like a world had unfolded in front of me. I was suddenly a mother, when had that happened? In what moment?

I looked at Cato, his eyes were open, wide and reflecting lights from the car window. His fingers were curled, grasping at the air. It made me think of Teddy, his eyes round as he waited for the moon, and I felt something like a weight press deep against me. This was permanent. This was real. I was bound to Cato by a deep sense of responsibility. My identity was no longer my own. It was as though I'd transformed without knowing it, and without any warning that I would be.

Parenthood was no longer just an idea. The months of worry about labour – it all felt small in comparison to the emotional weight of knowing that I had given birth to a new life.

The police have come at night.

There's been an incident with the Polish guy. The one who was quiet, but would giggle and sneer during the television ads.

He's sitting straight up on the gurney; his hands are in restraints. He isn't fighting.

A squad of police surround the bed. I think I see spots of blood on the floor.

We've been directed to stay on one side of the hallway. The workers are watching from the glass enclosure.

The residents look on; there is silence.

The returners seem to know what happened, but no one asks. Will says, 'Well, I'm not surprised.' And when I look the next morning, the floors are clean.

The time passes in a daze. Jenny leaves. She hugs each of us and gives me her leftover toothpaste. I am grateful.

I ask to be moved to a double room. The Olympics have started in Korea, and every time the ads and commentary start I can feel the others' eyes on me. I hear someone say the word 'spy', and I wonder if they think I'm a North Korean spy. 'Why's she always writing in her notebook?' I can feel eyes peering over my shoulder, and I start to write in small, cramped handwriting. Maybe they think I'm writing notes for the doctors.

'Ooh, she's cheating on her husband,' Tamyra crows during a television episode, she laughs and darts her eyes over to me.

I feel their eyes on me whenever there is an ad featuring an Asian woman. I start to hear footsteps behind me while I'm pacing the halls.

Or am I being paranoid?

Emma leans in to me. 'I spit out the pills,' she whispers. 'They're not going to get me that way.'

I have noticed the medication. I didn't before, except for the dry mouth. At night after the meds my eyes feel heavy and they close soon after lights out. My vision is starting to blur, I notice it when I'm writing, the words run together as though the ink is wet. I wonder if I should spit out my medication, but mine is liquid, so I take it instead.

*

'I want to change rooms,' I say to Shara, the one with curly hair and tired eyes, but who smiles no matter what. I have started to become nervous that when I open the door to my room, someone will be waiting inside.

'What, baby?' She doesn't look up from her phone.

'I want to change rooms, I want to share a room,' I say. I try to sound matter of fact and not paranoid.

'Why?' She looks up from texting.

'The others are talking about me, it makes me feel …' I wait for the right word '… uncomfortable.'

'Well, they might be talking about you, but it may be that they're jealous.' She looks at me; we are acknowledging what has been unspoken.

'I know,' I say. 'I understand that. But it's becoming too much.'

She nods at me. 'Remember, you can't control how others talk about you, but you can learn to stand up for yourself.'

I feel dejected, perhaps I won't be given a new room. However, an hour later, one of the workers shouts, 'Catherine,' and she gestures to the hallway.

I take that as my signal to change rooms. I gather up my possessions in my arms, my notebook, my jumpers and underwear, and I hustle to the hallway where another worker is waiting in front of my new room.

I can feel my memories sharpening. The days before the psychosis are still a blur, but my sense of who I am is coming back. It's slow and unsteady, but I feel more certain in myself. I can feel myself grounded in the present, being more aware of where I am, who I am. I find myself noticing the time, noticing the walls and the chipped paintwork. I feel claustrophobic; it's a slow suffocation.

I think more about the others in the ward. Do they feel the way I feel? They don't seem to question this place, like they are accustomed to the rhythm, to the waiting. We are all in this shared experience, but I wonder if they see it that way. I have a life outside, a good one. I have an identity besides the one that's been given to me here. As we sit together in the cafeteria, hunched over our plates in silence, I think about the way our paths have crossed and brought us here. If I saw Dave on the streets of New York, would I give him a second glance? Or would I cross the street to avoid him? Would I ever speak to Ali? Or Darren? Would I look at Tamyra and think that she's not a good mother? The last thought stings with recognition and shame. Who am I to say that? What would someone say if they saw me? I'm not a good mother.

James calls me a few times a day. Our conversations are becoming more normal as my sense of self returns. He is careful not to speak about what happened before, instead we talk about the mundane, what we ate that day, how we slept. James tells me about Cato. Cato is sleeping well, he's smiling more, he's learned to stay longer on his tummy without crying.

I talk to James while twirling the cord around my finger, aware of the clicking sounds on the phone. I know that we're being recorded. I keep the conversations short so as not to take up the phone line. I decide to ask James when I'll get to leave.

'Do you know when I'll get to go home?' I say.

'I really want you to come home,' he says with a sigh. 'But it's not up to me. It's up to the doctors. I've been talking to the doctor and she says that every time she sees you, you seem better.'

The doctor? I haven't been seeing a doctor. Have I? Oh, I realise, she must be watching me. I look over at the glass enclosure behind me. They are still looking down at their screens, shuffling papers. They seem to take no notice of me.

'Oh,' I say. I feel cold.

'Well,' I try to laugh. 'That's good to know.'

When I hang up with James, my mind is catching up. How have I been so slow? Of course I'm being watched. I'm a patient. They've been watching me all along. What am I supposed to do? What is supposed to happen? Am I acting in the correct way? Do I look sane? Should I not be writing in my notebook? I try to picture myself, viewing myself in a mirror. I'm neatly dressed, although I'm wearing a hoodie and pyjamas.

I wonder if I look too calm about being separated from my son. Shouldn't I be eager to go home? Shouldn't I be hysterical?

I decide to remain as calm as possible. 'The fastest way out of here is to act like you don't want to leave,' Will's words echo to me. I start to notice the workers looking at me. Their eyes following me as I walk by, as I pace. Are they texting about me? What are they saying? I try not to notice the eyes, the eyes that are watching.

I start to think of things I miss from home. Home is a place I can imagine. I picture it in my mind, our flat in London. The objects that didn't seem so special before now seem so dear. It's as though my sense of focus is expanding, the things that had been in shadow before are taking shape, and I am slowly becoming aware. Aware of something more than just the present moment. The medication in the plastic cups, the pacing in my blue foam slippers, the sound of the television.

I make a list of things I miss. I promise myself not to take them for granted again.

Hot showers
Tea with honey
Listening to the radio
A glass of red wine
Books
Walks around the city
Soft bedsheets
Holding hands with James

I know that I should miss Cato, but my mind is still blank when I think of him. Cato's name comes up in my notebook more as I'm writing. His absence feels palpable to me. Thinking of him is like trying to capture an echo.

I keep the pictures that James printed for me tucked in the back of my notebook. I keep them secret, I don't want the others to see. Every so often, I go to my room and look at them. I test myself by closing my eyes and trying to picture Cato's face. It doesn't work. I see nothing.

And so I open my eyes and look at the baby in the photos.

I still don't recognise him. I remember I thought that his eyes were like oceans, and I stare and stare at his eyes until his face becomes distorted and no longer looks human. I try to remember what it feels like to hold him in my arms, to remember what it sounds like when he cries. All I feel is blankness, no longing, no sadness, just the awareness that there is an absence. Maybe it's the medication, I think. In a way, it makes me feel grateful. Because even though I feel numb, I can sense that it's a wound, and I have no idea how deep it goes.

One of the photos is difficult to look at. I keep it behind the others because it makes me feel even more hollow. It's a photo of Cato and me, he is sleeping in my arms. The woman – me, I have to remind myself – looks eager and bright. There are tired smudges under my eyes, but my eyes are clear and my face looks like it's shining. In my arms, the baby leans against me, his eyes closed, his face is a curve.

I trace the scar on my stomach, thin and slightly curved, a ridge along my hipbone. It's the proof that Cato is real, that he did come from my body. I am a mother. I try to remember what it felt like to take care of another human being, but I can't imagine it now, it seems impossible.

When I leave this place, I will be with him. I don't know why, but instead of being comforting, the thought frightens me. The thought occurs to me that maybe I'm meant to be here. I'd never considered that before. Am I not sane? Even asking that question, doesn't it prove my sanity? I start to feel short of breath. This idea of who

I am, does that even exist? Am I real? I am real. I know I'm real. I take out my paper of truths, it's folded and creased now, the paper is rubbed smooth from where my fingers have traced the letters.

My talisman reminds me of the time that Leah took me to a fortune-teller. She said it was important because it was the year of the tiger, my year, which was inauspicious. She'd bought a charm for me on a gold chain, a medallion stamped with an ox. It would be a charm against misfortune, she said. I wore the necklace, where it stayed around my neck like a brand between my collarbones, the metal cool despite the humidity.

The fortune-teller was a thin man, balding with glasses. His office was in what seemed to be his flat, a large room lined by shelves of books. He had carefully taken out a piece of paper and had me write down my birth date. His English was broken, and so he spoke through Leah and gestured with his hands. 'Korean,' he said. 'Koreans are sad people.' He pointed to the TV in his room.

'Yes, Korean dramas,' I said. 'They are sad.'

He drew diagrams on the piece of paper, telling me which numbers to avoid. He told me that my elements were fire and earth. He told me to balance my yang, that I should be careful not to eat 'hot cold foods' like lychee or melon. He told me that I should never live by the water, that I should avoid the ocean. So I was not like my grandmother, I thought.

He looked at my palms and shook his head. 'Palms change,' he said. 'Destinies change.'

I thought he would tell me whether I would marry well or have many children. Instead, he closed his book firmly. He looked at Leah, who was fidgeting with her gold watch.

He looked me hard in the eyes, and I felt exposed, like he knew that I'd been crying the night before. I met his gaze, and he wrote a few characters on the piece of paper and told me in English to keep it with me always.

I wonder what he would say now.

My first days out of the hospital, I was focused fully on Cato. The weight of responsibility, it felt heavy. Each moment and action was focused on him and keeping him safe from harm, keeping him alive. I watched our apartment transform into a baby station, corners spilling over with scattered nappies and muslins. Cato's cries filled the rooms, there was nowhere to escape it. His screams were insistent and primal and drowned out all other thought.

Cato had no sense of night and day, and so we started to think of time in sets of tasks. Feed, change, sleep. Feed, change, sleep. It was sets of three, cycles that we had to repeat, again and again like military drills. We didn't have a chance to reflect or take anything in; when he slept, we waited and tried to re-energize, knowing that the cycle would begin again.

My only moment away from Cato was an hour I would take in the evenings after I fed him. I would hand Cato to James and escape to the bath, where I would soak in the hot water and close my eyes and dream of silence. That hour was precious, it was my time to be alone, to think, to remember that I had a self, that I was something more than a mother.

But more than a mother wasn't really accurate. I was a mother; I was still trying to figure out what that meant. Was it a full identity that encapsulated me? Was it a shadow that followed me? A word in parenthesis after my name? Was it something that I could slip on and off like a dress? I wasn't sure.

My identity, my existence had shifted without me realising it. The axis of my world had changed. Everything was now in relation to this other life.

'Hi, Mum,' the midwives would say to me on their visits. And I'd realise with a start that they were talking to me.

My sense of those days was exhaustion. The physicality of it erased my emotional senses. Why did no one talk about how tiring it was? Or had they, and I just hadn't been paying attention.

We did have moments of lightness. We read Cato nursery rhymes and wondered at his hands, his small feet. We took Cato with us to the pub, walking through the frigid air, smiling as strangers cooed at us, at this tiny baby wrapped in our arms.

My mother came over when Cato was a couple of weeks old. She flew in from Virginia and came to our apartment from Heathrow on her own. I remember that I was lying on the bed, while Cato was in the cot next to me. We heard a knock at the door, and my mother rushed into the room.

'Oh,' she gasped. She clapped her hands. Her delight was childlike and pure, and it made me feel like everything was worth it. She immediately settled in to make me seaweed soup so that I could regain my strength, and she scolded us for leaving the apartment and not staying indoors. Why wasn't I wearing socks? I should be keeping my body warm, she scolded. Didn't I know anything?

'Should I hang some peppers at the door?' I asked jokingly. She only laughed, but she watched me to make sure that I finished my seaweed soup.

She stayed for two weeks, taking over the night watch, sleeping on the floor next to Cato's cot to hand him to me when it was time for him to feed. She brushed away tears when she said bye to Cato, leaving him with a kiss on the forehead like a fairy godmother's blessing. When my mother left, my heart ached for her. Mother: I had a new understanding of the word.

Ever since I'd found out I was pregnant, I'd had the idea of taking a long trip to the US. It would be the perfect opportunity, I thought. James and I would share our parental leave, and we could see our family and friends. James was reluctant, but I was insistent, we'd never have this opportunity again, I said.

I had planned it perfectly and in detail. We would begin with a friend's wedding, make our way to James' family on the West Coast and then to Virginia to see my parents, and then to New Jersey to meet the rest of James' family and my friends from New York.

We would leave after Christmas, a few days before New Year's Eve. We still had time to spend in London, and I was determined to enjoy the moments we had with Cato. Before James went to work, I'd set up my seat on the sofa. I called it my 'battle station'. There were pillows, a tower of snacks, a large tumbler of water with a straw, an iPad, a phone charger, everything within arm's reach. And then I would settle in, strapped in to my breastfeeding pillow, with Cato lying on me, while I watched Netflix and breastfed. There were some days when James would come back from work and find me in the same position, unable to move because Cato had been feeding all day.

I didn't mind those hours while James was at work. There was something about sitting with Cato, it was like he was still tethered to me. I'd stare at him, at the curve of his cheek, and feel the warmth of his body against mine. I loved the way his mouth would turn upwards into a small smile when he was sleeping, and I would touch his eyelashes with one finger. He'd come from me. From my body, I'd think. It was a miracle.

I don't know if I'd describe what I felt as love, it was something beyond that. It was more primal, a fierce, possessive affection. He was ours. He was mine.

When James came home, he would sing as he held Cato, 'It's the three of us, Cato, Omma and Appa, the three of us are one family.' And it was true, it was the three of us.

When James' parents heard about my plan for a cross-country trip with the baby, they were particularly concerned. It unleashed a firestorm of text messages. It was dangerous to fly with a baby. It was dangerous to travel during flu season. It was dangerous to take him to a wedding where there was a crowd of people. How could we be so reckless? Didn't we care about the baby's health?

I was frustrated; it seemed so backward. 'If they think we're going to stay indoors for a hundred days, they're mistaken,' I said to James.

James agreed with me, but he had his own concerns about travelling to the US. 'You don't think it'll be too much?' he asked.

'No!' I said. 'It'll be great, it'll be so special for Cato to meet everyone. This is the one chance we'll have to do something like this.'

And because of my excitement, he reluctantly gave way.

As we boarded the plane to San Diego, I didn't feel any sense of foreboding, just expectation. They would understand, I thought. Once they saw him, our families would be glad that we came.

We landed in San Diego the day before New Year's Eve. The air felt expectant, rich with the smell of palm trees and coconut. We stayed in a resort off the coast. We were celebrating the wedding of two friends of mine from college who'd been together for twelve years.

Cato didn't notice the time change, and for once the jetlag didn't matter. Our cycle continued on. Feed, change, sleep. Feed, change, sleep. I expressed milk into plastic bags that I'd brought and kept them in a freezable lunchbox that James carried with him. At night in the hotel, Cato would scream and scream, and so I cradled him in my arms and sang lullabies until he fell asleep.

The theme of the wedding was a New Year's Eve party, the scent of salt water and freesias was in the air. I was a bridesmaid and I wore a dress lined in sequins with metallic thread. Cato was curled in my husband's arms like a snail, sleeping in the sling. We brought in the New Year in a cloud of confetti.

At the harbour, the groom sobbed through his vows, and we cried along with him. We danced with Cato in our arms. We cheered as we lit sparklers in the night, and the groomsmen hoisted chairs holding the bride and groom. Through the glitter, I thought of another evening, in another lifetime, in Hong Kong. That night on the balcony, looking for stars, things had seemed so hopeless. Why had I thought that that type of love was the only kind I deserved? I looked at Cato in my arms, his hands pressed against me, and I felt triumphant, a desperate feeling of love, of joy. I felt renewed.

I'd heard once that most of the cells in our body regenerate every seven to fifteen years, and so we become new, but with some parts deep within that will never be replaced. Still, it made me think of being a new creature, cleansed.

How lucky, we thought, that Cato got to witness this celebration, to bring in a new year of love. As we watched the bride and groom perform the tea ceremony, the bowing to their parents, the offerings to the ancestors, it also felt serendipitous. Cato was our lucky charm.

I am thinking of Cato's 100-day celebration. It was meant to take place by the water. James' mother had booked a seafood restaurant with a view of New York City. From the tables, you can see the ferries and boats go by.

We had ordered sticky rice cakes, boxes of fruits, a tower of red dates to represent abundance. Cato was going to wear a silk hanbok, dark blue and pink with embroidered gold lettering. I'd spent an afternoon at a New Jersey party store looking at the sparkling balloons and party hats. I'd bought colourful paper bunting, streamers of ribbons, straws with pineapples on them, emoji stickers for the party favours. It all seems so superficial now – the scraps of plastic and paper.

Thinking of the party, I feel a deep sense of guilt. What were we celebrating? Had I tempted the fates by being too reckless? My grandmother would have been stern with me – when you have something precious, something to rejoice in, you hide away, everyone knew that. I had been too careless, too loud in my happiness, and now we were all being punished. It was the balancing.

Even in the ward, I can't escape my feelings of guilt.

'Catherine?'

I'm colouring with Darren. He's working on a picture of a leopard, and I have one of a unicorn.

It's Christine, the social worker. Everyone knows who she is. Whenever she leaves the glass enclosure, she's immediately trailed by residents. They follow her from room to room; 'Christine, Christine,' they call. She ignores them. She usually looks frazzled.

She looks nervous now.

'Come with me,' she says, and I follow her into the activity room. I can feel the eyes of the others following me.

Christine is wearing a crocheted pink beanie, and she bites her lip when she talks to me.

I try to remember to act naturally. I sit carefully, but then I pause, no, I shouldn't sit too carefully, I don't want to seem posed. Will she be able to decide when I get to leave? Or is it just the doctors?

I try to picture what I must look like, with my glasses and carefully tied hair and hoodie. She has a binder next to her. I wonder what it says about me.

We sit and look at one another. She doesn't meet my eyes completely; she looks beyond them.

'So,' she says. She smiles at me.

I smile back, but not too widely. We could be two people sitting for a business meeting.

'How are you feeling?'

'Good,' I say. 'I feel good.'

She starts to flip through the binder. 'Your husband provided a lot of paperwork for us. He's been very ...' she pauses, 'involved.'

I smile. 'That's his personality,' I say. 'He's very thorough.' I wonder what exactly he's provided for them. I see his annotations and notes in the margins.

She nods. 'Do you have any questions for me?' she asks.

I want to ask when I can leave, but I think of Will's words, and so I start with another question first.

'I want to know what meds I'm on,' I say.

'OK, so looking at your file, you're on haloperidol and Benadryl.'

I've never heard of haloperidol.

'Haloperidol is an antipsychotic.' Christine seems to guess my thoughts.

'Benadryl?' I ask.

'I think it's to shut down your milk production,' she says. She says it without emotion.

She waits for me to say something.

'I want to know when I can leave,' I say. The room seems to change, I feel Christine stiffen, but I try to look nonchalant.

'When do you think you'll be able to leave?' she asks.

'I'm not sure,' I say. 'I think it's up to the doctors.' I remember at the end to phrase it as a question.

Christine immediately waves her hands.

'Oh, but it's not up to the doctors! It's up to you, it's up to us working together as a team. Your husband, me, you, we're all a team, so we're going to work on it together,' she says. I'm not sure what that means, but I try to stay calm.

Our meeting is interrupted by Dave, who is slamming his wheelchair against the door. 'I need to speak to you!' he says. 'I see you've been discussing things with my paralegal, but it's time for you to talk to me.' Christine sighs.

She nods at me. I realise that I've been dismissed. And then what?

I pace the hallways, trying to breathe.

I am still pacing, back and forth along the corridors, when Will comes up to me. He's wearing faded sweatpants and a patched hoodie.

'You saw Christine,' he says.

He looks at me kindly. I think he's going to make a joke, or maybe tell me I've got it easy compared to him, when he's so desperate to stay. Instead he smiles.

'I have an apple in my room, if you want one,' he says.

I recognise the care of the gesture. I nod. 'Thank you,' I say.

He half-jogs to his room and returns with an apple in his hand.

One of the workers is frowning after him.

'Here,' he says. 'Don't worry, they won't care as long as you don't eat it in front of the others.'

It's tart and slightly warm, but it reminds me of sunshine.

Will looks at me appraisingly. 'You'll be all right,' he says. 'You got people.'

Yes, I think, I do.

And as I savour the apple, I think of James, and the evenings when I was pregnant, sitting at the kitchen table cutting apples together, the peel unfurling like a globe. We'd talk about the future, with hope, with expectation. Everything had seemed within our reach, just like the apples in our hands.

What am I doing here? I want to be home. I want to be with James. I want to be with Cato. The yearning is so sharp I want to collapse, to sit on the floor and weep. Will is watching me, a sympathetic half-smile on his face. But I don't weep.

Instead, I think of the hidden star in the apple in my hands. Teddy and I would clap our hands when my mother cut the fruit horizontally to reveal it. To think, a star had been waiting, just for us.

After San Diego, the next stop on our US trip was LA. We arrived there when fires were raging across the landscape. It was New Year's Day. James' older brother, Matt, lived in a suburb in a beautiful house made of white stone that had been constructed a year before. 'You go in and you pick out what house you want,' Matt had said.

Each house in the subdivision was a variation on the model houses at the entrance. Their house had swooping ceilings and everything was white: the furniture, the linen, the floors, the kitchen island. It felt beautiful, if sterile. The neighbourhood was an unending reflection of white – white box houses that had the same doors and windows with a fingertip of space separating them.

My brother-in-law is a doctor. He has the type of charm that's loud, brash, full of swagger.

His wife is a nurse, tall and pretty with a soft voice. Her name is Grace, but James and I call her Hyung-soo-nim, meaning 'older brother's wife', the 'nim' signifying honour. I knew they didn't think that we should have been travelling with a baby. 'You should eat some seaweed soup,' my sister-in-law said as a greeting.

James' aunt threw a New Year's party for us. The house was full of cousins, aunts and uncles, the West Coast side of James' family clan. We drank rice cake soup and ate sticky sesame cakes for good luck.

I met James' grandfather for the first time. He was 102 years old, with white hair and faded eyes. His eyes reminded me of James' eyes, and they had the same smile. He was sitting at the table with a bowl of rice cake soup.

'Grandfather,' James said.

His grandfather turned to us. I could tell he was confused for a moment, and I wondered how he felt, all these children running around the house. But he smiled at us and stroked Cato's cheek, and he looked at me as though he recognised me from a distant past. We held his hands, and Cato reached for his cheek.

After dinner, we lined up according to age and bowed to James' grandfather for good fortune in the New Year. First James' aunts and uncles, and then the cousins, and then finally the cousins' children. Each time, he smiled and waved his hands over us, as his descendants came to him in waves. We walked to him and pressed our foreheads to the ground. I felt my head touch the floor, and I thought of all the generations who had done this for centuries before.

James' grandfather pressed dollar bills into the children's hands, shaking his head when they tried to refuse. It made me think of my grandmother. She would always put money into my hands when we left her house, and my mother would make me give it back, only for us to find it tucked into my pockets later. 'Buy something to eat,' my grandmother would say.

As we left, James' grandfather waved at us, beaming.

We spent our days in a coffee shop across the road from Matt's house. James was still working remotely, and so he was logging on to his computer and drawing up plans for research, talking with his students. Matt and Grace left early in the mornings for their work shifts. We didn't have a car, so we walked each morning along the highway to the coffee shop. We sat in the courtyard, while James worked over a cup of coffee. I had Cato strapped to me, breathing in the California sun. Cato would snore, his face pressed against my body. I'd look down and I could see his cheek pressed against me, his fist a tight curl against my skin.

When the sun started to get too hot, we would go back to the house; the white was cool, a refuge from the heat. I was still breastfeeding, but I developed thrush, so I walked around the house with my shirt around my waist, airing out my breasts to get rid of it.

We would later find out that the entire house was Nest Cammed, with motion detector audio and visual surveillance cameras. 'It's a California thing,' Matt said. He said it was for home security. James was furious, but I could only laugh. It made me nervous, though, and I started to notice the blinking of lights in the corners, cameras in the rafters. I started to monitor what I said to James, I felt like we were being watched.

On our third day, I developed mastitis, an infection because of blocked milk ducts in the breast, and so I became bedbound with Cato next to me. The cure to mastitis was to keep breastfeeding, so I kept him close. He was again my fellow inmate. I felt trapped in the white room, unable to leave because I couldn't fasten my clothes without feeling pain. Cato didn't seem to mind; he didn't cry, instead he slept soundly, his cheek pressed against the white sheets. I'd lie on my side and shiver because of the fever, and I'd watch him sleep. I'd trace the lines of his eyes, the curve of his cheek, his dark hair in the sun.

Time didn't seem to matter anymore, Cato was either feeding or not feeding, and I'd slip in and out of consciousness. James would bring ice water, the ice cubes would dissolve in the heat, and I'd stare at the white walls and wonder how much time had passed. I'd whisper stories to Cato and sing him the songs I remembered, the ones about a mockingbird and diamond rings, and the Korean one about elephants and blue moons, and I'd watch as his eyes would crinkle, and I'd let him wrap his hand around my finger and marvel at the strength of his grip.

James tried to shut off the camera monitors, but it was a complicated procedure, and he ended up covering as many as he could with pieces of white paper.

At night, James and Cato would sleep, but I would lie awake. I started to hear the sound of the cameras whirring.

In the fairy tale of Shim Chung, after Shim Chung decides to sell herself as a sacrifice to the sea god, she lies to her blind father, telling him that she is going away. She cries silently and makes sure that he can't feel the wet of tears on her cheek.

The sea is stormy, and the fishermen tie an anchor around Shim Chung's feet so that she will sink quickly, a merciful death instead of struggle. There is lightning, thunder, the waves come fast and hard, and she is thrown overboard.

But then, a miracle. She finds herself in the underwater sea kingdom, and she is crowned queen. Queen of the sea, with pearls like tears around her neck.

I always wondered about this fairy tale, that moment before being thrown into the sea. I believe she has tears, but I think it's only because she won't see her father again. She has surrendered to the fates, and she feels triumphant in her sacrifice.

The divers in Korea are always women. They swim along the coast, diving to deep depths without any breathing equipment. They ignore the dangers of the strong currents, providing for their families by collecting abalone from the sea floor. I wonder if they think of Shim Chung as they dive deep beneath the waves. I used to imagine they'd find pearls, pearls like tears, gifts from the queen of the sea.

We arrived in Virginia during a blizzard.

I had been apprehensive about Virginia. Mostly because I wasn't sure what to expect when we saw my father. When James had texted a photo of Cato to announce our son had been born, my father had texted back, 'OK.'

I couldn't imagine my father with a baby. Would he be distant? Would he be irritated by Cato's crying?

We stepped up to the front door. My mother opened it and embraced me.

My father was standing behind her, hesitant. I saw his face, he looked eager.

'Here,' I said and held Cato out to him.

'Ah,' he said. He reached out his arms and held Cato close, his glasses slipped off his nose, he was face to face with him. And then he smiled a full smile.

'Hello,' he said, as though Cato was an adult. My father took Cato to the piano and played the opening notes of a Bach prelude. For the rest of our time in Virginia, if Cato wasn't feeding, he was in my father's arms.

My ever-thrifty parents had transformed a large cardboard box into Cato's cot. My father had drawn cartoon characters, slightly wobbly Disney faces and Hägar the Horrible. It made me remember my father in restaurants drawing lines on napkins with a fountain pen, while we watched as the lines transformed into cartoon faces. I hadn't thought of that memory for years.

We took Cato on walks in the woods, through the park area where the snow was falling in banks and drifts. He looked up in wonder, at the light shining through the trees, at the grey of the sky, the pattern of the leaves, and I thought what he must feel – looking at the world turned around.

We spent those few weeks in silence, even Cato seemed to know that it was a quiet house. He didn't cry much during the day, but at night he refused to sleep and I'd stay awake with him curled next to me in the bed, the two of us, silently listening to the creaking of the walls, the sounds of night. He'd cry quietly into my shoulder, and I'd try to soothe him to sleep.

My father would knock on my door each morning and take Cato from me so that I could have a few more hours of sleep. I would come downstairs, and my father would be lying on the couch, with Cato sleeping on top of him. Cato's head was tucked against my father's chin, and his cheek was pressed against my father's chest. My father was gazing at the ceiling, his arms curled around Cato. They were still; separate from the world.

It made me wonder at how my father must have held Teddy and me when we were small. What had changed? What had gone wrong?

Teddy came to Virginia to meet Cato. His hair brushed his shoulders, and he looked more like my mother's son than ever. I had to erase the memory of a dimple-cheeked boy who would follow me around. He was uncertain around Cato, and patted him gingerly with one hand, as though he was afraid Cato would break.

I realised that my family expected me to act a certain way as a mother. 'You can't do whatever you want now,' my mother said to me sternly when I told her that I wanted to leave the house. 'You have to think of Ji-hoon.' She always called him by his Korean name.

Yes, I did think of Cato. I thought of Cato every moment. 'You shouldn't even be here,' my mother scolded, but she said it while smiling, I knew she was happy to see Cato. She sighed. 'What must your in-laws think.'

'Catherine?'

It's one of the doctors from behind the glass enclosure. I am in the TV room writing in my notebook. I follow her into the cafeteria. I try to be calm. Maybe I can leave.

She is slight with dark hair. She has glasses that slip off her nose. I notice that the rest of her face is blurred.

'So,' she says. 'I know you spoke to Christine.'

Her hands are fidgeting, and she's looking past me at the clock behind my shoulder.

'How're you feeling?' she asks.

'I feel good,' I say.

I see her look at me appraisingly. Maybe she can tell that I can't make out her face.

'You've been very unwell,' she says.

'Are you sleeping?' she asks.

I nod. She is watching me. I try not to fidget.

'I'd like to know how I can go home,' I say. I try not to sound eager; I try to sound measured.

She waits for me to keep talking, and even though I want to, I don't. I wait.

'Well,' she says finally. 'Only you know when you're ready to go home.'

'I don't understand what that means,' I say.

'It means exactly what it sounds like. We've spoken to your husband, he feels like you're still not completely yourself.'

My annoyance shows.

'He's a perfectionist,' I say. 'I feel fine, I'm basically a hundred per cent.'

But I've said it too forcefully, I can tell.

'Don't worry, Catherine, it's about how you feel, not someone else's perception of how you feel. We listen to you.'

I sit back. She isn't listening.

'Are you eager to leave?' she asks.

Of course, I think. Of course. Not too eager. I pause carefully. 'I miss my family and would like to go home.'

'Well, let's wait another day or two, let's see how you feel.'

I force myself to smile calmly. 'Great,' I say.

What does it mean that James doesn't think I'm myself? I can't remember what it feels like to be myself before all of this, whatever it means. I am feeling something like rage, but a dampened one. Somewhere there's an emotion, but I'm only feeling the echo of it. I'm suffocating in this place, trapped within these hallways of repeating walls. Does James not trust me? Does he think I should stay here? I feel helpless; I want to scream. But I don't.

I want to use the phone, I want to call James, but when I lift the phone, there is no dial tone. The phone is heavy in my hand. It's not phone time. So instead, I pace. Back and forth, my slippers are soft against the linoleum floor. I try to time my breathing with each footstep, a few counts for each breath, in and out, I am trying to remember to keep the inhales as long as the exhales, no panic, just deep breaths that fill my body with air.

Inhale. Exhale. When I breathe this way, it reminds me of diving. I learned to dive while I was living in Hong Kong. I wanted a feeling of control. I had always been afraid of the ocean, it was too vast, too open, but I wanted to feel lost, with only my breath to guide me.

The first time I went diving, staring at the horizon, I remember I thought of Shim Chung. I'd been loaded down with metal weights to make sure that I wouldn't float. 'Beginners tend to go to the top,' the instructor had told me. 'Stay down.'

The water was choppy and the boat was tossing with each high wave. The instructors promised that underneath the water it would be calm; it was just the surface that was broken.

I fell backwards into the water, and as I felt myself sink, and the cold rush over me, I tried to remember to take deep breaths. It was like counting steps. Being under the water, it was so calm. It reminded me of the calm before a thunderstorm, so still, and so silent. We went deeper and deeper, clutching the rocks to keep from being pulled into the deep sea by the current.

I tried to sway back and forth with the current, keeping an eye on my oxygen. I looked out into the deep blue, the expanse of darkness, and I felt a sense of terror, of emptiness. And even though I desperately wanted to go back up to the sunlight, away from the blindness of the deep, I forced myself to stay down, watching the glimmer of light be swallowed by the ocean.

We are watching the Olympics. It's the ski jumping.

Haru is upset because his show is on. '*Criminal Intent*. Channel 28,' he says. He's wearing furry slippers and a bathrobe that's slipping off his shoulders. He looks like an old man from a comic book.

'No,' Will says. His legs are crossed on the couch and he's munching on an apple. He's been in his room all day but has come out for the Olympics. '*Criminal Intent* is on every single day, Haru. The Olympics are once every four years. Four years, Haru!'

Haru looks at the worker in the room; it's Tim, a slight man with a thick accent and a buzz cut. Tim shrugs.

'Haru, no one wants to watch your stupid show,' Will says. 'Majority rules.' Tamyra laughs. She has tissues sticking out of her ears because she says she has an earache.

Haru looks on the verge of angry tears. He turns and stomps to the glass enclosure.

'Oh great,' Will says. 'Now he's going to tell.'

Emma looks apologetic. 'He watched *Criminal Intent* this morning. I remember.' Emma took her medication today, at least that's what she told me. I can tell because her eyes are glassy, and she's stopped talking so quickly. Instead, she's slumped on the couch, her papers lying forgotten next to her. I try giving her a smile, but she looks past me, as though she can't focus, and she leans back against the cushions.

Mick is sitting in his wheelchair by the door, his back is straight, he still has the posture of a military man, and he's rubbing his hands against his shaved head. He turns to Ali. 'Who do you root for when you watch this stuff?' Ali has his eyes closed, he has Vaporub around his nose, and he's taking deep, slow breaths. I vaguely remember hearing that VapoRub helps with panic attacks, and I wonder if that's why I haven't seen him walking the halls today. Ali opens his eyes and raises an eyebrow. 'USA … obviously.'

Mick shrugs.

Sitting next to me is a new woman. I haven't seen her before. She has dark hair and she hasn't told anyone her name yet. She's huddled and shivering, she has her sleeves pulled over her hands.

We watch the Olympics in silence. I notice that the woman next to me is crying.

Tamyra is talking to her boyfriend. She sees me waiting and glares at me. I shrug and take a step back. When she hangs up, I notice that she's blinking away tears. She lingers by the phone, I ignore her and dial James' number, a reverse-charge call.

'Hello darling,' he says.

'Hi,' I say. I take a breath. We are being recorded. I wonder if James knows. I hear the familiar clicks in the background.

'I talked to the doctor,' I say.

'Oh yes?' He sounds eager. 'What did she say? Did she say you were going to be released?'

'Well,' I say. 'She says that you don't think I'm a hundred per cent yet.' I try to keep any accusation from my tone. 'So, I don't know, I think I have to wait awhile.'

There's a silence. And when he speaks, he speaks slowly.

'But, Cat, you aren't a hundred per cent, I thought you knew that.'

I keep my voice light. 'I feel basically a hundred per cent.' Out of the corner of my eye, I see Tamyra watching me, I turn so that my back is to her.

'You aren't, you're different, and that's fine, but you're not yourself yet.' He pauses. 'You don't even ask me how Cato is doing. It's like he doesn't exist. I think it's going to take time, maybe months, or even a year.'

'I don't have a year,' I snap. 'I want to leave here … I can get better when I go home. I'm ready to go home.'

'I know,' he says. 'And I want you home. I told you, it's not up to me.'

'It's OK,' I say. James doesn't know. I feel like I'm caught in a reflection of the world, and there isn't a way out.

I push aside what he says about Cato. Why can't he understand? It's like Cato doesn't exist? I am in a deep sleep, cocooned to the truth. Even in my numbness, I recognise this fact. This is how you survive as a ghost, I realise. This is how you exist; this is how you surrender. Around me, all I can hear is the sound of the television, the murmur of the workers behind the glass enclosure. I feel like howling, I want to shatter the glass, hold the shards up in my palm.

We arrived in New Jersey on a grey day. We'd been travelling for thirty-one days, from San Diego to Los Angeles to Virginia and then finally to New Jersey.

I was exhausted. We took the Amtrak train, carrying our bags from Washington DC. On the train, I thought I'd lost our backpack with our passports and a journal that we'd been keeping since the start of our relationship. James was wearing Cato in a sling, and he jumped off the train to look for the bag. I heard the train doors close.

'Come back!' I shouted, but James gestured to me. 'I'll see you in New Jersey!'

'Get on the train!' I ran to the conductor, screaming hysterically. 'You have to let my husband on board, he has a baby, I need them on the train!' I saw James sprinting to the front of the train and, miraculously, the doors opened.

'What were you thinking?' I said. 'You don't even have any milk, and I have the tickets.' James shrugged and smiled at me. My heart was pounding. I must have looked like a madwoman.

'It's all fine,' James said. 'It'll all be fine.'

I was on hold with the lost and found at Union Station when we found the backpack. It had been under the seat. I laughed wildly in relief. This was the moment when I realised that the trip had taken more out of me than I'd expected. The sleep deprivation, the constant moving around, everything felt exaggerated. The colours of the world were too vibrant. I felt a breath away from weeping.

I was relieved to have reached our final destination. I felt triumphant; we had made it.

My in-laws' house was in a New Jersey subdivision with matching roofs and windows and backyards of trees. It was quiet except for the buzz of highways. New Jersey made me feel uneasy, it reminded me of the scenes from the movies with identical rows of houses and strip malls that were too bright.

My mother-in-law embraced me when we arrived. 'Welcome, you are finally home,' she said. And I believed it. Even though it was February, there was still tinsel on the walls from Christmas, and we settled in to one of the upstairs rooms.

We had only been in the house for a few hours when I realised something didn't feel right. I could hear a noise, a tinny buzzing and beeps that sounded like monitors. 'I feel like we're being watched,' I said to James.

'Hm?'

'Do your parents have cameras too?'

'No,' he said, 'I don't think so. Don't worry, I'll check.'

My father-in-law had installed a Purell machine in the house because of the flu season, and each time we came in from outside, he wanted us to gel our hands. It reminded me of the hospital announcement that was on repeat in the maternity ward: 'Please gel your hands. Please gel your hands.' I could hear the voice, a chorus in my head, echoing.

My father-in-law and mother-in-law started to talk about Cato, concerned about the effects of travel on a baby so young. My father-in-law checked Cato's temperature with a thermometer and worriedly counted his fingers and toes, as though he might have lost one on the way. 'We've planned a 100-day celebration,' my mother-in-law said. 'But don't let anyone hold the baby or get too close, it's flu season you know.'

'When I had my first baby, I didn't leave the house for four months,' she said. 'And no one was allowed to visit. Why did you let so many people hold the baby in California? Each time you posted a photo of someone holding him, your father-in-law would get so scared... What if they'd dropped him?' And then she told me the story of a baby who'd been dropped at a celebration party and died.

'Don't worry,' I said. I tried my best to assuage their fears and address each comment, but it was as though I was speaking into a void. The questions and worries didn't stop.

Why was Cato so big? We must not be exercising him enough because we'd always been travelling. Why wasn't he rolling yet? Didn't we know that he should be rolling by now? It must be all the travel. Why did we hold him in a sling? It must be affecting his body, his limbs would grow crooked. Why did he cry so much? He must be stressed because of all the travel. Why wasn't he sleeping through the night? It must be all the time changes and the travel. Was he coughing? Was he sick? Did he have a temperature?

Each comment and criticism, although kindly meant, stuck at me like pinpricks of a needle. Was I such a terrible mother? Was I doing everything wrong?

I already knew the story of James' uncle, the firstborn son of James' grandfather, who had smiled so widely when he met me. His firstborn son had died when a pot of hot soup fell on him. I told myself that this was why my parents-in-law were cautious, but I started to doubt my own instincts.

'Should you be feeding him again?' my mother-in-law said. 'You shouldn't overfeed him, he's too big!'

'Well, actually, I'm meant to be feeding on demand.'

'You should feed him with a bottle, then I can help you. Why don't you bring a bottle? Do you have any? I want to feed him.'

I tried to explain that I needed to feed because of my mastitis. This was waved away. 'If you feed with a bottle, you can pay attention to how much they're eating. Look, he's so big, he can't even move around!'

And so I started apologising whenever I took Cato away to be fed.

'Why are you holding him? He needs to learn to sit on his own, put him in the swing, don't hold him. You hold him too much.' Cato would scream and scream, and I would stand hovering over him, my whole body leaning towards him but not able to reach out. Whenever I tried to express concern, my mother-in-law would laugh, exaggerated laughs, and then her eyes would dart towards me. Why was she laughing? I didn't understand.

'Have you gelled your hands? It's flu season, you know,' my father-in-law would say nervously, and then my mother-in-law would laugh again, while gesturing to me to gel my hands. I saw myself as if through a camera lens, rubbing my hands together under the Purell machine. I could feel the sting of the alcohol on my palms.

'Maybe we shouldn't have come,' I said to James. 'We seem to be causing them a lot of stress. I'm doing everything wrong.'

'Don't worry,' James sighed. 'I knew this was going to be difficult. But don't think about how they think of you. You're fine. They just worry, that's all.'

My mother-in-law talked excitedly about the 100-day celebration. It was happening in two weeks. All of James' New York clan was coming. My parents were going to drive up, and I heard that my sister-in-law was flying in from California. I felt excited, but the idea of so many people was exhausting. A hundred days, I thought. A hundered days, and Cato would be safe.

It was on the fifth day that I decided I had to leave the house for a few hours away. I was tired of being indoors; I wanted to move. I was starting to feel trapped, I felt like I couldn't take breaths, but my decision was met with concern. 'But it's so cold outside, you shouldn't take Cato outside when it's so cold. He could get the flu.'

'There's a state flu epidemic right now, you can't take him to a crowded area, he could get the flu and die.'

'We can drive you, but you can't take public transportation, it's so crowded in there. If he gets the flu he'll need a spinal tap, it's very dangerous for babies his age.' My father-in-law's face was furrowed.

'If you want to go, you should go, if you're happy we're happy,' my mother-in-law said. She smiled and laughed while clapping her hands, but she was glancing at me with a look of warning.

What did she want me to do?

I ended up deciding to stay in the house, just to stop the chorus of caution.

Cato screamed often, it was as though he could sense the tension. The house was kept to a high temperature, in line with the Korean tradition that mother and baby should be kept warm. It made me feel even more compressed, like I was being bound.

I started being unable to sleep at night, my in-laws' voices were repeating refrains in my head, and I'd cry out of frustration. My tears were hot, and I'd wipe them with the palms of my hands while I fed Cato, trying to keep them from falling on his cheek. I felt helpless and enraged, but confused and doubting. Maybe I was a terrible mother. Maybe I was being irresponsible by travelling when Cato was so young.

Why had we left home? Why hadn't I listened? What would I do if Cato became ill? I felt like I was in the labour ward again, except this time I wasn't trusted to take care of my son. More than lost, I felt guilt. Guilt for not having listened, guilt for endangering my son, guilt for not being an obedient daughter. I was being split between the role of daughter-in-law and mother.

I had been selfish to make this trip. I hadn't thought about Cato. I hadn't thought about James' family and their anxieties. In my sleepless state, I went over their worries in my mind. What if someone had dropped Cato? What if he'd got sick from the plane? What if? What if?

And then there was the constant feeling of being watched, of being monitored.

James found out that his parents had installed Nest Cams in their house as well. It linked to mobile phones, and both of James' brothers had access to the audio and visual feed. James was so enraged, he tore the main camera out of the wall.

'Why didn't you tell us there was a camera?' he said.

I must have looked panicked because James' mother said, 'Why are you so worried, Cat, no one is listening to what you're saying. No one cares.' Then she laughed with her eyes darting.

Yes, and that was the problem. No one did care. No one was listening. My words meant nothing in this house, in this whirlwind of noise. I was a blind man's daughter in a deaf man's house – I said this to James. And no one was listening to me. No one was speaking my language.

'You're doing great,' James told me. 'We're doing great, look at Cato, he's healthy, he's happy.'

'Are we not doing the right thing? Is Cato OK?' I asked.

James waved his hands, brushing my concerns aside. He was irritated by his parents, but he didn't seem concerned by the running commentary or the constant questions and criticisms. He just ignored it; it was as though nothing was being said. 'Don't worry about them,' he said. 'They don't mean what they say.' But I couldn't stop listening.

And it wasn't completely true. His parents *did* mean what they said; however, what I only slowly began to realise was that they didn't mean their words to be taken seriously. They were used to speaking without being heard. Words were just sounds, not carefully chosen.

I started to become paranoid that James' mother was signalling to me in a language separate from the rest of the family's. Her exaggerated laughing motions, her darting eyes. They didn't match her words, and I didn't understand. What was she saying to me? What did she mean? Why couldn't James see?

'You just have to surrender!' James' mother would say frequently, throwing her hands up in the air. 'That's the only way to survive being a mother!' And I'd know it was kindly meant, but each time it felt like a pressing of hands against me, a suffocation. Surrender. I was meant to be a sacrifice.

I started to feel the weight of duty on me. I wanted to leave, to escape, but I knew that was impossible. We were bound.

I also sensed that with Cato's birth, James' mother felt that her son had fully left and now had another family. I saw it in the way she looked at us, the way her body leaned towards James, the flash of her eyes when James came into the room to hug Cato and me first. 'Before you know it, he'll grow up, and he won't want to spend time with you. He'll leave,' she said, and I sensed the note of bitterness there. There is a Korean expression that love only flows down, like a river or tears, love flows from one generation to the next, never the other way. I tried to imagine what it would be like to have Cato grown up, married, starting a family, leaving me behind. I thought of James and his mother; instead of a line, we were creating circles. In my future, I saw James' mother, standing on the other side, reflected towards me.

It had been a week since we arrived in New Jersey, and I finally insisted that we needed to leave the house and go to the city. We would take Cato. 'We have to go,' I said to James. 'Even if they're worried, I need to go.'

'Don't worry what they think,' James shrugged. He seemed unbothered, even when his mother tucked antibacterial wipes in our bag, and his father asked us to check Cato's temperature every few hours.

We trudged onto the New York bus system, James carrying the pushchair, I had Cato tucked into a sling. For the first time since we arrived in New Jersey, he slept soundly. He was curled in my arms, and I could feel his heartbeat, his breath on my skin. As we walked through Manhattan, I felt like I was letting off a burden of air. I cried in relief at being able to breathe, at being anonymous in this city of faces. No one was looking at me, I felt safe in the blizzard of snow and people.

We returned home in the evening; James' parents had been waiting up for us. I could tell from their faces that they'd been anxious. I stayed awake that night listening to their murmurs.

The next morning, James' father sat with me. He poured coffee for me, and we sat facing each other at the glass table. He gave me a smile, and I could sense that we were about to have a serious conversation.

'Does James treat you well?'

'Yes,' I said.

'OK, good. I know that having a new baby, this is difficult.' He paused. 'Have you heard of post-partum depression?'

'Yes,' I said. And then I realised, he thought I was depressed.

'It's very common,' he said. 'Eighty-five per cent of women have it after they have a baby. I think you might have depression.'

He spoke kindly, his face was grave.

'I notice that you are worried all the time, that you aren't sleeping, this is dangerous, you need to take care of yourself. I think we are making you feel anxious. I get worried, I worry a lot, and I know I speak roughly. I don't mean to.'

I started to cry. His diagnosis of what was happening was so accurate. He could see so clearly what was going on. He knew.

'I have three sons,' he said. 'Of my three, James, he is the most difficult, but he is also the one with the most conviction. You once told me …' and he quoted to me the conversation we had the first time we met. 'You told me that you wanted a husband with kindness and conviction.

He has both. And I know that he loves you. And I believe that you are a strong woman, you will get through this.'

I looked at him, and I saw his hands shake, and I saw his face, and then I realised what had been happening, what I hadn't seen in my state of worry and fear. My father-in-law wasn't worried because of our actions; his anxiety was his own. I saw a man who had seen so many worst-case scenarios, who felt powerless to help and was terrified of having to recognise those signs in the ones he loved. He knew he was an anxious man, he knew that he was always worried, it wasn't Cato he was trying to protect, it was himself.

I started to feel like I could breathe.

He smiled at me, but then he ended the conversation with his usual tic, the worst-case scenario. 'In most cases, post-partum depression is not serious, but you have to be careful. Because I had a patient who shook her baby. She shook him and then the baby went blind.'

And my breath caught in my throat.

Koreans say that in the moment between sleep and waking, if you wake, paralysed and unable to breathe or shout, a ghost is sitting on your chest.

I remember being terrified of this feeling. Being awake, frozen and not able to move. I'd open my mouth to let out a silent scream, and I'd think of the ghost on my chest. Where had it come from? I'd imagine that it was a ghost from generations ago, the ghosts of my grandparents' dreams, the ones that had been taken from them. Ghosts of the past, of lives interrupted, of expectation, of yearning. A heavy burden, passed down for me to hold.

After my conversation with my father-in-law, I went back upstairs.

I started to feel as though the air was stiffening. I felt my chest clench, and I had trouble taking in a breath. The ground shifted suddenly, like someone had given a quick shake to the world. I went to feed Cato, holding him close, but then I noticed that my hands were clutching him tightly. Would I suffocate him? Was I holding him too close? His eyes were darting at me. James' eyes, his mother's eyes, they were looking at me with fear.

Was I going to shake him? Would I blind him? Was he afraid of me?

I tried to put the thought from my mind. It was the feeling that I sometimes got of vertigo, of looking over the edge of a tall building and imagining the fall.

My mother-in-law called for me.

'Cat!' she said. She wanted to talk about Cato's 100-day celebration that was happening in a few days.

'A lot of people are talking … There's a lot of drama going on behind the scenes, believe me,' she said.

I nodded. I could hear their murmurs in my head.

'And don't worry, at the 100-day celebration, I'll watch people to make sure they don't drop the baby,' she said. 'I'll watch very closely.'

'But,' I said, starting to feel my chest tighten, 'maybe by watching, you'll make people nervous and then they will drop him.' I thought of the vertigo, the fall, I thought of Leah looking nervously at our balcony when we moved in to the new apartment and looking over the edge. The same fear when dreading something, that anticipation, does it make the event inevitable?

At that moment, James' father came into the room. James' mother made a laughing motion, while her eyes darted to me.

And then I saw my mother-in-law as well. Her criticisms, her worries, they weren't because of me. They were because of her own family, and she was doing her best to manage them. And I, I was the problem, I was the one messing it up, by ignoring her cues. She had been asking me to mirror her, to look carefree, all the while her words were a warning, and her body language was to reassure my father-in-law, so that he wouldn't have to worry. Her laughter, it was a pantomime for his benefit, a habit developed in a deaf man's house, to make everything look as though it were running smoothly. Just like the silence my brother and I had grown up in.

Her darting eyes were her tell, her nerves when things weren't going smoothly as she had planned.

Of course, my father-in-law knew what was going on, he knew that there was something at the core of the house, something untrue, something to diagnose.

While this was obvious to James and his brothers, to me it was a hard-won conclusion. I couldn't have come to it any other way than consuming every lie, every presumption, until all that was left was the truth. In my mother-in-law, I saw a portrait of contradictions. A woman who loved adventure and had the spirit of a young girl, put into a box of traditional marriage and family. Her family was her centre, her axiom, and she loved her husband. She had to follow a dictated path or break completely. She'd chosen to adapt, and her constant phrase, 'I surrender', it was the truth. She'd chosen to surrender, to accept her fate, her happiness. Her son, my husband, was the only one who shared her love of adventure, but he had left her behind, going to London, away from the network of family that she knew and loved.

In James' father, I saw James, but an extreme version. A man of knowledge and wisdom and kindness, who'd been taken over by fear after years of seeing worst-case scenarios. His sense of powerlessness as a doctor caused him to see signs of potential dangers in the everyday, a new dimension ruled by illness and worry. It led him to embrace religion and faith, and he could sense that, biblically, his three sons weren't following the path he was hoping for them.

And James, like in the fairy tales, the third son, treasured, chosen, loved, was destined to be apart from the other two brothers who were lost in the woods, the only one to emerge. Underneath his happy childhood, I saw a new dimension of darkness to his stories. A constant reminder of mortality, of illness, of seeing symptoms, a reminder of not being in control, a force that shaped my husband into a man of principles and clear thinking, always methodical, always in control. A man who turned away from faith and superstition, who chose to believe only in what was proven, what was evidential.

'I fell in love with you at first conversation,' he'd said, and I finally understood what he meant. In his family, full of love and noise, no one was actually listening. There was too much going on, too many voices and opinions. Noise.

And then, even though I didn't feel like it, I mirrored my mother-in-law and made an exaggerated laughing motion.

It was like I'd been sprinting, and this was the moment when everything came to a sudden stop. The world flipped. Everything changed, but nothing had changed.

I believe this was the moment that ultimately triggered my psychosis. I processed all these things in the single moment that my father-in-law and mother-in-law looked at me and our eyes met. And I saw us, apart from time, our portraits, our mirroring actions. We were all existing, but out of sync with one another, repeating the patterns of the past.

Koreans believe in reincarnation, in recurrence, souls that are reborn again and again.

When my uncle's son was born, he was born with a mind like a kaleidoscope; he doesn't speak, but communicates through drawings and dance, living between worlds. My grandmother had blamed herself. A fortune-teller had once told her not to mourn her unborn son, the one who had died in her womb. He will be born again, she said, as your grandson. And so my grandmother had wished, had waited. And then, when my uncle's son was born, she thought, the living incarnation of her dead son, of course he wouldn't belong to the land of the living. She was being punished for questioning the fates – for wishing too much.

I wonder whether James' grandmother had looked for her eldest son in the eyes of her grandsons. His name would have shared a character with James' grandfather's name, and his father before, a wish traced back generations, a wish interrupted.

I think that perhaps, even though they fear it, Koreans wish for recurrence. They yearn, and they wait. They live like ghosts. They wish for the past to become their present.

I went back upstairs and tried to catch my breath. Everything would be fine now, I'd figured it out. But I felt like I'd downloaded too much information, and I was still processing, catching up.

Three sons, diagnoses, mirroring actions, darting eyes.

I looked at Cato sleeping peacefully in his cot. I wanted to hold him, and I leaned over to pick him up, but then his eyes opened. And then it happened.

His eyes turned to devils' eyes. Dark eyes with flashing red pupils. A flash, and then his eyes, James' eyes, James' mother's eyes, darted towards me with fear.

I tried breathing again, but my breaths were becoming short. The walls felt thicker. I hadn't understood the expression about walls closing in, but it felt like they were now.

'James,' I gasped.

He came into the room, and I saw his eyes widen when he saw my face.

I told him that we needed to leave the house. Now.

'I can't breathe,' I said to him. 'Please trust me. I need to leave.'

He paused.

'I need to leave now.'

'OK,' he said. 'OK, let's leave.'

I felt a window opening in my mind: we were going to leave. We would be fine. I'd thought that leaving the house was impossible, but James had just opened a door.

'Can I pack?' he asked. 'Would it be OK for me to pack our things so that we can go?'

'Yes, yes,' I said. I started gasping and sobbing. 'I need you to look at me straight on,' I said. 'I need you to not look at me like I'm crazy or I'm going to fall apart, I swear.' His eyes were still trusting, they were still all right, but I didn't know what I would do if James' eyes changed too.

'I need you to repeat exactly what I say, word for word,' I said. I needed to know that he would understand me completely, that there would be no more misunderstandings. No more side languages, I needed to know that we were all speaking the same language, on the same plane.

'Yes, he said. 'I will repeat exactly what you say.'

'Word for word,' I said.

'Word for word.'

Cato was crying quietly, and so I picked him up, but I didn't look at his eyes. I sat on the bed holding him while James packed our things methodically. There was a question I remember from middle school: who would you trust to pack your parachute? And I always knew, when I met James, that he would be the one I would trust.

He was talking to himself as he laid out each of our things and separated them. Somehow, he packed all our bags within minutes. It was as though he'd been prepared all along to escape at any moment.

And then I had a thought. James and his bag, the one he always had. I'd teased him for never being without his backpack, but maybe there'd been a reason he was always ready to leave, always ready to escape. Was this his childhood? One that was claustrophobic from stress and anxiety? He used to tell me that some of his happiest memories were walking into town alone, spending the day walking to the drugstore, reading comic books. And

I saw another dimension to that story; I'd never thought to ask why he'd left the house, why he wanted to be alone, but I realised that it was a reminder to himself that he was in control.

'We're going to go to a hotel,' he said. 'Unless you want to go back to London?'

'No, no,' I said. 'I'll be fine, there's no need to over-correct. I just need to get out of this house.'

He nodded.

'Repeat, please,' I begged.

'OK,' he said. 'There's no need to over-correct. You just need to get out of the house.'

He thought for a moment, and then he took out his phone and booked a hotel, one that was a few minutes away.

I felt the weight, that weight lifting from my chest. I didn't look at Cato, I didn't dare, but I felt him shuffle in my arms. What did it mean that his eyes had changed? What was happening?

But it was going to be all right now. We were leaving, it had seemed impossible, but we were doing it. Generations of duty and obedience, and we were leaving. Just like that. Could my grandmother feel this? This liberation? We were leaving in a stream of ribbons, we were escaping this loop, this repeating pattern of mothers and sons, of fear. I thought of James' mother's story of her brother who had died from hot soup falling on him, of my mother trapped in her in-laws' house. We would break this pattern.

I could hear James' parents downstairs. I heard them speaking to one another.

'I can't see your parents,' I said, the weight was back again. I started to gasp, the walls were closing in again, I was becoming trapped again, we were going to stay in this loop, this loop, loop, repeating loop.

'You can't see my parents,' he said. 'OK.'

He rushed downstairs, and I heard him speak to his parents. The front door opened, and I heard them leave the house and drive away.

'What'd you say to them?' I asked.

'Don't worry about it,' he said.

'No, I need you to be honest with me. I need you to tell me,' I said. 'I need to know that you believe me. That you trust me.'

'I just told them that we need to leave and that I needed them to leave the house for a while.'

I started to breathe again. I could feel Cato against me, his heartbeat, it would be fine, we would get out of this.

I didn't know what was happening to me, but it was as though the world was being shaken fiercely like a snow globe, and I was the only one who had a sense of balance. I was holding on to James as hard as I could, I needed him to believe me, to reassure me that I was still in reality. Maybe I was having a panic attack, maybe I was just dreaming, I couldn't be sure, why was the world compressing?

James loaded the spare car, the one with duct-taped windows and boot.

He took Cato from me, and I noticed that my hands were shaking. I still couldn't look at Cato. I was running away, away from the house, away from this place.

I sat in the front seat and tried to concentrate on breathing. The houses were repeating, the same versions of neighbourhoods, and I started thinking about what Matt had said about his house. The repeating houses. And I thought of *A Wrinkle in Time* and the description of the houses and the children bouncing balls in sync with each other in the driveways. Would we ever be able to

170

escape? Were we just staying in the same moment? In the same place?

We finally passed the town centre and I was still gasping for breath. I expected the sky to suddenly open.

When we got to the hotel, James said to let him check in. I sat with Cato on the patterned couch in the lobby, counting my breaths, hoping that the world would stop shaking. Two Korean men in suits approached me. 'We're looking for my phone,' one of them said in Korean.

Were they? A thought flashed through my head. Were they friends of James' parents? Were we under surveillance? What if word got back to James' family that we had been seen at a hotel? Would they be able to deal with the scandal?

The hotel looked like a seedy hotel from the movies, with red carpeting and textured red walls. I thought I could hear the thrum of surveillance cameras. Were we being watched? I imagined a room of screens, and our images multiplied.

We were being tracked, I thought. What if people were looking at my Instagram, at my Facebook, and analysing everything we were doing? I was friends with James' cousins on Facebook, is that what my mother-in-law meant, was that what she was warning me about when she said people were talking? My hands shook as I deleted my Facebook and Instagram apps. I decided to delete my WhatsApp history as well. They were watching us.

'What are you doing?' James asked. He looked at me. He was holding the room key.

'I'm deleting everything,' I said. 'I just need some time to myself.'

He nodded slowly.

As we walked down the red corridors, I thought I could hear murmuring from the other rooms, from behind the doors. I heard the buzz of cameras in the corners. 'I've always wanted to stay here,' James said.

I tried to nod. In my arms, Cato was stirring; I glanced down at him. His eyes were devils' eyes.

My room-mate Liz is blonde and in her forties. She spends her time shivering in her bed, only emerging for mealtimes, which she shuffles to with a yawn, rubbing her eyes.

She has a book next to her bed, *A Tree Grows in Brooklyn*. I ask her if I can borrow it.

'Sure,' she says, but her eyes narrow. I can tell that I've broken a rule. Personal belongings are off limits.

'Just for a second,' I say quickly. 'It's one of my favourites.'

'I've heard it's good, I haven't really had much time to read it.'

There is a bookmark on the second page. I thumb through the pages. It's miraculously clean and unmarked, when everything in the ward is worn through.

She asks me to read out loud. My voice is shaky, the words are skipping off the page in my vision, but for a moment we are both on the fire escape of a tenement building in New York.

'That was nice,' she says.

'Thank you for letting me read,' I say.

I try something tonight. I hold the liquid and pill in my mouth; I don't swallow them. I walk quickly to my room, and I spit into the sink.

I want to feel. I don't want to fall asleep in a fog, I want to know what's happening.

Around me, I sense the mood in the ward changing as everyone settles down, calm, sedated. The pace slows, people stop talking so much, there's the sound of the television and then, one by one, we pad along to our rooms to sleep. I'm one of the last, but I follow along. Step, step, one two, one two. Above us, the fluorescent lighting hums.

For a moment, I remember pacing in the labour ward with Cato in my arms, singing him songs that my grandmother used to sing. I remember the sound of the lights, the press of his body against mine, the promise of morning. I press my arms crossed against my heart, there's a sharp ache in my chest, and I'm trying to stop it.

Lights are out in the ward.

I can hear Liz snoring.

The room is dank and a small dresser in the corner is making strange shadows. My bedframe is metal, I can feel its bones sticking through the mattress. The bedsheets are thin and rough; they scratch my skin. It's dark, but there are angles of light coming in from the doors. From far away I hear screaming and the faint sound of footsteps. I hear the doors opening and closing.

I feel empty, and from deep within I feel a sense of yearning. I turn to my side, I almost expect to see Cato in a plastic cot next to me, swaddled in his hospital blanket. I wonder if he realises I'm gone. The thought makes me feel nauseated. I hope he doesn't realise, it's better that he forgets. I try to picture Cato's face, but I can't, I only see his eyes, James' eyes, James' mother's eyes.

I hear my mother-in-law's voice, what was it that she'd always say? 'I surrender.' Should I surrender to my thoughts? I don't think I can, whatever that might mean.

I feel compressed, I think of the locks on the doors, the heaviness of the doors. I try to count my breaths slowly, and I want to think of home, but I can't.

Instead, I think of my grandfather's compound in Korea and the summers I spent there as a child. The compound was built on the side of a hill, with a campus and church lined with bamboo groves. At the top of the hill was a house made of red brick.

In the summer heat, the house was stifling. We would stay indoors, standing in front of the air conditioning unit playing chess with the African stone pieces which were cool in our hands. At twilight, we would run in the backyard amongst the black marble tombstones. The names on the stones were written in Korean, the graves were empty, they represented the parents that my grandparents had left behind in North Korea.

We'd lie on the cool marble, pressing our cheeks against the chiselled stone. I could hear the sound of my heartbeat against it, echoing against the rock.

We'd play in the shadows until it became night.

I think of this now, as I count my heartbeat in the ward. The dark is like glass, bright splinters of light from the hallway in our room. And I think of my ancestors, who were a mystery to me. I didn't know their stories. My only link to them is in my DNA, in the shape of my hands, the reflection of my eyes. What did they feel? What did they imagine? Had this happened before? It felt so familiar, pre-written somehow.

And nearby in a dark like this one, James and Cato are sleeping. Away from me. But along the same line of the globe. I think of my great-aunt, who always slept with her feet pointed north, in the direction of where she longed to be. She had left her husband and son in the north; her son had just learned to walk. They were separated in a moment of fate, never to be reunited. My great-aunt never forgave herself; why had she insisted on travelling ahead, she should have waited. She died without remarrying; she thought each day might be the day that they'd meet again. They would meet again, she said. She knew it. She only worried that her son wouldn't recognise her with her white hair.

I think of love, my fascination with love stories, and my grandmother's warning. I used to think her warning was about men like Drew, the violence, the cruelty, the emotion parading as love, but I think it was a warning against something purer. She meant what she said. It was a warning against the triumph of love, because something so beautiful, so raw, can only end. To bare one's heart is to know suffering, vulnerability. It is a destructive force.

That's what makes it beautiful, to know mortality and failure, but to step off the edge anyway.

When we arrived at the hotel room, I immediately wanted to leave. It was all wrong, the walls were too red, they were humming. There were plastic flowers gasping to live, there was a television screen that was a shadow in the corner. I could hear whispers from the hallway. My breath felt uneven again.

James started to unpack the bags.

'Please sleep,' he begged me. 'I just want you to get some rest. And then we can talk.'

I shook my head. 'No.' I couldn't sleep. I couldn't stay in this room.

'I can't!' I shouted. Around me the patterns on the wall were running, scampering across the red. The room was spinning, but only we were standing still. I thought I could see figures running, running as fast as they could out of the room. I felt trapped, I was on a balcony again, and I wanted to leap. Couldn't James see what the stakes were? The world was shaking, and somehow I needed to escape, to walk, to be away from the suffocating feeling. I felt like the walls were turning and turning, that I was stuck in a mirror of reflecting images, of reflecting lives. I didn't want to tell James about Cato's eyes, because I didn't know what I would do if James looked at me with fear as well.

I tried to take a deep breath. James was watching me.

'I need to call Teddy,' I said. 'He will understand.'

And he would understand, I thought. He was the only one that could. I knew that he saw me for me. Not as a mother. Not as a wife. Just Catherine. Noona.

I took my phone and went into the bathroom to call Teddy. It was 5 a.m. in Seattle, but he picked up the phone. 'Hi, Noona.'

'Teddy,' I said.

My breaths were coming in gasps. He waited.

'I can't breathe, Teddy,' I said. 'I don't know what's happening. Something's really wrong. Everything is closing in, I'm not sure what's happening, but it feels like everything is strange, almost like it's all happened before.'

There was a pause.

'Do you know what I mean?'

'Yes.'

'What do you do when you have that feeling?' I said.

'Well, mostly, you have to find a reason to laugh. You have to find it absurd.'

'I'm trying to laugh,' I said. 'But it just feels too serious. Too dark. I'm not sure what's real.'

'OK,' he said. I knew that with Teddy, I had to wait. I looked at myself in the bathroom mirror, I looked the same, like normal.

'Noona, just be calm. Where are you right now?'

'I'm in a hotel with James ... and Cato,' I said.

'In a hotel?'

The words tumbled out of me, as I told him that we'd left James' parents' house, that James had done the impossible thing and got us out of there, he'd broken the rules of duty and obedience, we had done the impossible, I'd been a blind man's daughter in a deaf man's house, and we had done the impossible, but something, something was still wrong.

'Noona, can I talk to James?' Teddy asked.

James was sitting on the bed worriedly with Cato. He looked at me with tired eyes, but they were still his eyes, they were still trusting.

'It's Teddy,' I said.

James handed Cato to me and left the room. I sat with my head leaning against Cato's, I could feel his breath warm against my cheek. His skin was soft, softer than powder; he was still trusting, still leaning against me.

James came back into the room, he handed me the phone. He gave me a half-smile.

'Noona,' Teddy said. 'I think you need to sleep. I know that when I don't sleep, it really affects my thinking.'

'Yes,' I said, 'I agree, but I can't sleep right now, I need to breathe, I need to walk. I can't breathe in this room!' I could hear my voice in my head, I was sounding desperate.

'OK, Noona, just be calm. You'll be fine. Just listen to James. Whatever he says, just listen to James.'

I pictured Teddy as a child, a small boy, my foxhole buddy.

'You know, Teddy, you were always my foxhole buddy.'

He laughed. 'I know, you're right. Noona, you'll be OK.'

I hung up the phone and looked at James. He looked weary and uncertain.

I wanted to see Teddy, I wanted to ask him to fly here, to remind me that everything would be OK. 'Maybe Teddy should come,' James said to me, as if he knew what I was thinking.

'No,' I said. 'No, don't bother him.'

James tried to smile at me. 'If you can't sleep, why don't we go on a tour of my hometown,' he said. It was something we'd talked about, his childhood, and how if we'd met in high school, he'd have taken me on a high-school date. 'Why don't we go on a high-school date,' he said. 'We can take Cato.'

Yes, I thought. Yes, we could do this. I could do this. Leaving the room felt like a test, but we stepped out into the hall, and I could feel my heart, a closed fist in my chest.

I immediately felt relieved; this was going to be fine. I was going to be fine. We packed Cato carefully into the car; he looked at me innocently, his eyes had no hint of the devilishness that they had before. He cooed at me, and I smiled back at him. We would be fine. James drove, and I stayed in the backseat next to Cato with my hand on his leg. We drove down the streets of Tenafly, past the bagel shops, the delis and diners.

We parked the car on a side street and took Cato out in the pushchair.

James led me to the drugstore where he used to read comic books. 'I used to come here all the time when I was a kid,' he said. He smiled, but he looked exhausted as we walked in. 'Let's buy some supplies,' he said. He was moving slowly as though in a dream. Perhaps he felt the weight of what we had done, I thought. Perhaps he felt the weight of leaving.

As he stood by the shelves, I looked at James carefully. I noticed that he had eczema on his face and hands. He pulled out an inhaler; he never had to use one in London, but after a few days in New Jersey, his asthma had returned. He took a deep breath with the inhaler. 'I used to spend hours here,' he said. And I suddenly saw him as a young boy with an oversized backpack, finding silence in the drugstore aisle, with chapped lips and shaggy hair, away from noise, away from diagnoses.

The colours in the pharmacy started to feel too bright. What was happening? I could feel the walls moving, closing, pulsing.

I started to see demons' faces in the drugstore aisles, an older woman with a walking frame stared at me, and her face was distorted. One eye was bulging out of her face, the eye socket was open, no eyelid, and her nose was long and hooked. What was happening? I couldn't tell if it was my imagination. I started to look around the drugstore shelves, the boxes seemed like they were pulsing too, the colours were vibrant, too vibrant. The words on the pharmacy signs were flashing at me. 'Relief', 'Pain', 'Escape'. What was going on? Was I dreaming?

I looked at James, he was still focused on the supplies, he didn't seem to notice what was happening. He moved slowly towards me and smiled at me again. I could feel my breath constricting. 'I need to go back to the hotel,' I said.

'OK,' he said. He looked relieved. 'Let's sleep, I'm exhausted. I think Cato is exhausted too.' I looked at Cato sleeping peacefully in his pushchair. And then I realised: Cato, I'd forgotten about him.

We left the drugstore without buying anything. I walked quickly to the doorway. It was pouring rain. The sky was dark. There hadn't been any thunder or lightning, no warning, just torrents. When did this happen? The rain was dark; it was pelting the ground.

'What should we do?' I asked. I could feel the eyes of the old woman staring at me behind us. She sounded like she was trying to talk to me. I ignored her.

James didn't seem to notice the rain. He stood hesitantly. 'Let's just go,' he said, and he took out an umbrella from underneath the pushchair. We walked slowly, sheltering the pushchair and trying to make sure that Cato wouldn't get wet. As we walked to the car, I wondered whether this was a dream. Was this a test? Should we wait out the storm? How would James' father feel if his anxiety caused us to leave the house, I wondered, only for us to die in an accident? It would be his version of hell, I thought.

James took a deep breath before he started the car.

In the car, I saw the sharp blurs of lightning and started counting, but I couldn't hear the thunder. It was raining so hard, there was only the sound of the rain. I started counting my breaths instead, I could feel Cato's breathing in the car seat next to me. His eyes were closed; he was peaceful. I could feel James' concentrating, he was trying his hardest. The rain was coming down faster so we could only see the headlights of the cars ahead. I thought of the quote from the Charlie Brown comic, 'Security is the feeling of being in the backseat of the car, while your parents are driving.' And I thought, if I were to die at this moment, I had a sense of peace. Cato's hands were grasping my finger. We were safe. I trusted James, I knew that he would get us back safely.

I felt like I was floating, calm. 'I feel like we escaped something,' James said as we walked into the lobby.

'Yes,' I said. The hotel lobby was wrong; I felt it like a jolt going through my body. It was crowded with people, so many people, and they were all turning their heads to look at me. Why were they looking at me? As I walked through them, they were pushing into me, jostling me. Some of them had distorted faces like the woman in the drugstore, some of them smiled at me with shining eyes, and then there was Cato's face in the crowd, but twisted into a demon's face, with a disfigured mouth and dancing eyes.

I shut my eyes. What was this trick? I refused to believe it. I held on to James' arm, and when we were in front of the hotel room, I ran in and closed the door. The room sounded like it was breathing.

James was exhausted, but he changed Cato, gave him to me and sat by me as I fed him. Cato was quiet; I tried not to look at him, but every time I did, his devil eyes would dart at me. I closed my eyes.

'What's wrong?' James asked.

'Nothing,' I said quickly.

We closed the heavy curtains. James put Cato in the cot, and he and I lay in bed. I tried to sleep. My mind was racing. Next to me, I could hear James snoring, and I heard Cato's steady breath. I just need to make it to morning, I thought. Morning will be a new day. The old world just needs to be destroyed in order for a new one, you have to break the walls to build them anew, I thought.

I'm not sure if I slept then, but the next moment, my eyes were open, and I heard a voice.

It was a voice in my head, my own voice, but it spoke with clarity and strength. Each time it spoke, the room filled with light. Where was the light? The curtains were still drawn. There was a darkness in the room, but the light was trying to fight. Somehow, I felt instinctively, I knew it was the voice of God. I felt his presence in the lights, in the dawn.

I immediately felt a sense of calm.

'God?'

'Your son needs to die.' The voice was simple, straightforward. The light was shining dimly now, but I could sense it fighting.

'What?' I felt panic taking over my body. 'Please, no, please.'

'Are you trying to bargain?'

'No, I'm not trying to bargain.' I started to cry. I felt helpless. What did this mean? What was happening? I didn't understand, I thought we were going to be safe, I thought we had made it. We had done the impossible thing, we'd left the house, I thought that was the test, that was all there was. What if I did bargain? It wasn't under my control, none of this was in my control. I didn't know how to make this nightmare, this dream, stop. I decided to let go. If this was the cost of my happiness, I would accept it.

'I accept it,' I said. 'If this is what's going to happen, I accept it. I accept.' I was shaking, terrified, but then I felt darkness come over me. And I felt nothingness, like a hand had been pressed over my face and smothered me. And then there was a dim light, and I could hear the sound of Cato breathing, it sounded steady, but then it stopped, and there was just the sound of the room. And somehow I knew, even without looking at him, that he had passed.

I prayed. I hadn't prayed since I was a child. Faith was something I'd felt before, something I'd sensed, omnipresent, like a shadow, but it wasn't something I'd chased since then. I prayed for mercy. I prayed to not be afraid anymore. I just wanted to stop fighting, to accept. I started to hear Cato breathing again, he was back, he was back. I felt the light, cool and delicate, and then I felt darkness, the smothering again. And I woke up again, this time I was face down, pressed against the bed.

The voice was in my head again. 'Your son has to die, and it has to be your husband's fault.'

'That will break him,' I said. I thought of James' grandfather, who was responsible for the soup falling on his son's head. He'd had to live with the guilt of his firstborn son's death. He was 102 now, so many years to live with the guilt. James, the infallible optimist, how would he survive?

'Yes, it will break him, but it will make him stronger. You need to be there to support him. You are his Beatrice.'

And then the voice was gone, I sensed a finality in its statement. Beatrice, I was James' Beatrice. So James was Dante. I had a thought. Did that mean we were in Hell? Had we died in the car driving in the storm and woken up in Hell? How many circles of Hell would we have to travel to reach the end?

I lay awake and thought of the evidence of the past day. What was the darkness? What were the demons? The distorted faces? Was I dreaming? Was I dead? Was I in Hell? Was this why I couldn't sleep? Was this why I felt the darkness pressing like hands against me?

I started to think further, past this day, and I started to see the patterns, fairy tales, the story of three brothers, East and West, the baby who was dropped at a celebration and died. The baby who died when a pot of soup fell on him. James' father the deaf man, my father the blind man. James' mother a reflection of me, Cato, growing up to be like James, and in the centre, throughout it all, James, James and me, me and James.

It was strangely exhilarating to see these patterns, like putting together a story when there were only pieces before. And through my dread and my fear, I saw the beauty in them, the patterns in the universe. I could tell it was dangerous, this raw energy, this coursing feeling, and for a moment, I wished I could tumble in, tumble into the madness. I felt like I'd caught a glimpse of another dimension, of the void, of the truth, of possibility. This feeling was beautiful; it was terrifying. I would never be able to harness it, I knew, I would never be able to control it.

I felt like Icarus, gasping in what was awesome, transcending fear.

Because suddenly, I wasn't afraid. It wasn't in my control, I wasn't in control. I surrender, I thought. And when

I surrendered, I felt invincible, because when I looked beyond fear, beyond the terror, all I could see was love. My love for James, my love for Cato. That was love, it belonged above, higher than any force. Was this what my grandmother was warning me about? The force that was love, and I would only know loss.

I tried to imagine losing Cato, I knew it was going to happen. I couldn't imagine the searing pain of it. The despair. The love as a destroyer. I would need to be there for James.

The next moment, I heard James wake beside me. He smiled, his eyes tired, and he looked at me with concern.

'Did you sleep at all?' he asked.

'I did,' I said. 'Actually, I'm not sure,' I said truthfully. I saw James' smile disappear as he watched me. His eyes were searching mine; his eyes didn't look trusting anymore.

'Oh, Cat,' James said. I was no longer in bed, I was standing outside of it, striding around the room. I felt powerful; by surrendering, I had won. I was going to hurt today, I was going to lose, but I was ready, I had accepted it. I was ready to leap.

James looked at me worriedly. 'Cat,' he said. Perhaps I'd been talking out loud. I could feel my body emanating energy, emanating light. I was glowing; I was alive. I wanted to be outside, to feel the wind, to scream.

'I need to talk to Teddy,' I said. 'I need to talk to Teddy.' I needed to explain to someone who would listen. James was starting to look panicked, and I didn't want to scare him.

'I want to go out,' I said. 'I want to leave this room.'

'No,' James said. 'We're going to stay here. I want us to talk. I want to know what's going on.'

'There's nothing to say,' I said. 'Let's not over-correct.'

The suffocating feeling was back. And then James was pacing the hotel room, back and forth, back and forth across the red carpet.

'Cat,' James said. 'I think I should call my parents, because I need them to take care of Cato. I want you to get some sleep today.'

I nodded, anything to help James. His voice was echoing, it was echoing, this wasn't right.

'Will you let me call them?' he asked.

I nodded again.

He stepped out of the room. I noticed he took Cato with him.

I called Teddy. The conversation was scrambled, but I remember telling him that everything would be OK. I was Beatrice, I didn't know what that meant for now, but I knew that I was Beatrice, and it was my responsibility to get us out of here.

'Do you remember?' I asked. 'Do you remember being a kid and flying kites?'

'Yes,' he said.

'Don't be scared,' I said to him. 'You're going to go on a long trip, Teddy. You're going to go around the world.' There was silence, as I described the trip he'd already taken a couple of years before, but this Teddy didn't know about it. This was another life, a version he didn't know.

Then, a small voice, I could hear him crying. 'OK, Noona,' he said.

'You're going to go to so many places! You're going to sell all your stuff, and you're going to take a tent and a backpack and walk,' I said. 'And you're going to grow your hair, it's going to be so long, longer than mine.'

'OK, Noona,' he said, I could tell he was trying to stop crying. 'Whatever James says, you do it. He's going to take care of you. You'll be OK.'

There's a rush of newcomers on the ward. Will says it's because it's Valentine's Day. I'm not sure what that means.

There's Persephone, a woman in her fifties with a bright blonde wig. She's a self-proclaimed psychic. She giggles and laughs like the ward is a newfound delight. 'Oh what fun!' she says about everything. She loves my slippers, she wants a pair, but they ran out a long time ago. I tell her I claimed mine from the bin.

I wonder if the newcomers are involuntary like me. I can't tell if they want to be here or if they want to leave. The newcomers appear without any fanfare, they just show up suddenly in the cafeteria, in the TV room. Some of them greet Tamyra and Will with an indifferent familiarity, as though it's expected that they are meeting again. There's never any formal introduction made, I guess the workers are too busy. We learn their names piecemeal, and some don't bother introducing themselves at all.

One of the newcomers is a Korean girl who scurries. She has a Bible under her arm, and she keeps her head bowed. She looks like she wants to say something to me, but when she sees me talking to Tamyra, she closes her mouth and walks away.

Then there's Lorena, a pretty college student with piercings along her ears. She comes in wearing a hospital robe; she has thick cotton bandages around her wrists. She moves hesitantly, like a sparrow. It occurs to me that she looks like prey. Dave barks at her and guffaws when she jumps. She sits next to me gratefully in the TV room as though she's found safety.

'What's it like here?' she asks me.

I'm not sure how to answer. What would be the right answer? I'm aware that the workers are listening.

'It's OK,' I say. 'Everyone is nice.'

'Do you feel safe here?' she asks. I see Tamyra roll her eyes.

'Yes, yes, I do.' I know that she's scared, and I wish I could think of another way to reassure her. Just be smart, I think. Don't ask questions like these. Be aware.

And then, 'Why are you here?' she asks. And everyone pauses, both workers look up from their phones.

I stammer. 'I … I got sick,' I say. 'I have a baby, and then, well, I was travelling, and I got sick. I was having a lot of stress from my husband's family, and I couldn't sleep.' The words tumble. How can I explain? I'm not sure where to begin.

'Let's watch the damn Olympics,' says Tamyra. I smile at her gratefully. She doesn't smile back.

In the hotel, time bent. I started to see things multiply, my sense of reality was fragmented, it was like I was forming memories that would duplicate, but each with a slight variation.

I saw James pacing the hotel room. Cato was in his arms.

I saw James pacing the hotel room in a loop.

I saw him shaking with our son's dead body in his arms.

I saw him again and again, with the same result: our son, dead.

Copy paste copy paste copy paste. Forced to walk around the hotel room in an infinite loop, trying to keep his son alive, but failing. My body on the hotel room bed. I saw this, hundreds of times, smaller and smaller images, like thumbnails on a computer screen, a miniature James, pacing and pacing, shaking while holding Cato in his arms.

I couldn't scream, I couldn't move, I had my hands over my ears, over my eyes, I wanted to stop seeing it. I wanted to stop living it. But here we were, living it again and again.

I could hear James' parents in the hallway. In the hallway of red wallpaper.

James rushed out with Cato in his arms, and I started screaming. 'I know, I know,' I screamed. 'We've failed. We are in your version of Hell.' I saw James' mother's face lined with worry, her eyes still darting, his father's face, his arms reaching out to me.

Somewhere James was shouting, I could feel him grab my shoulders, to pull me back into the room. He was sobbing. 'No, no. Just leave, just leave.'

He shut the door, but I could still see them standing in the red hallway, as though I was watching a screen projection. My mother-in-law was holding Cato close.

I was fracturing, I was splitting into versions.

And then like someone had pressed fast forward in my brain, I skipped ahead: James was crying in the car. 'We're going to the hospital,' he said. He was speaking quickly; he kissed me. And then he smiled, and I saw that boy at the wedding, the one who had thrown a rope to me, who had seen me and pulled me in. 'You trust me?' he asked.

I said, 'Yes, I trust you.'

As he drove, I saw our lives again and again: meeting at a wedding, meeting at a party, at a library, on the street. I saw us jumping off cliffs together, I saw us grow old, I saw glimpses. We'd lived them all, we'd always met, we had always fallen in love, but it always ended here. In the same place, in this car park, in front of the hospital. Yet again.

James kissed me fiercely. 'Let's go,' he said.

As we entered the hospital, I had the feeling of being on a set. There was a crewman holding a light, and someone walking by with cameras. Ah, I thought, I understand. This was a set, designed by Hell, a set to take the place of Purgatory. The receptionist was a demon, with ink-dark eyes and a twisted, pointy face. She winked at me. Her eyes danced with merriment.

James was standing by the desk, filling in paperwork.

'OK, what do I need to do?' I said loudly. 'This was very good, but how do I break his reality?' I addressed the demons around me, the ones sitting in the chairs, the ones holding their arms in bandages, the girl who was staring at me without blinking.

James shushed me.

I sat down. We were never going to be seen, this hospital was a set. We were in Purgatory, and James didn't realise. We were never going to be seen. We would be here for all eternity.

I tried to think about how to escape it. How did I help James? I was Beatrice, I needed to be the one to guide him, to guide him through the circles of Hell, but what was I meant to do? I tried to find a voice in my head, but there wasn't one. Perhaps I was meant to exit, perhaps I was meant to restart, so that we could begin again and do better the next time. I needed to exit. I thought of the possibilities, where could I go? How could I do it? But I looked at James, sitting wearily, his face furrowed as he typed messages into his phone. His phone kept buzzing. I needed to exit so that we could restart, but I wasn't going to leave without him. I looked over at the reception desk, the nurse winked at me again.

James' lips were chapped. I realised then that he hadn't eaten or drunk anything since the morning.

I took his phone and threw it to see if I could get his attention.

The girl who'd been staring at me picked it up silently and handed the phone back to him. 'Cat,' James said. 'Please,' his tone was gentle. 'Please sit.'

The room was spinning, time was passing too quickly, it was all happening at once, each moment pulsing with energy. I collapsed at his feet; I could no longer stand. I could hear James shouting, 'Could I get some help please? Someone please help me. Please.'

'Someone help him,' I screamed. 'Why is no one helping him?'

I started to pull at my clothes and scream. I pulled my hair as hard as I could. Maybe if I hurt myself, maybe if I did this, I could break James' reality. I could show him that we were in Purgatory. That we needed to exit. I felt the demons rush towards me, their faces pressing in gleefully, and their hands pressing on me as they twisted my ankle and pulled me down.

I fought and screamed. I fought with all my might, with flailing arms. I scratched, I bit, I kicked. I heard James shouting somewhere beyond me. I felt the hands pull me down to Hell. What would happen to me? I had failed. I had failed James. The nurse receptionist's face was there, she was winking at me and laughing.

And I suddenly had the thought of an insane asylum. I realised this was my fate, as though it had happened already, my fate was to be committed in an insane asylum for all of eternity. There were clamps on my wrists. I heard James' voice in the distance as though through a tunnel. I tried to strangle a demon nurse with her nametag, I thought of James' mother, perhaps she had been through this before. 'I surrender,' I screamed.

I remember lights, bright ones. I saw an operating table, I saw demons standing over me, licking their lips and clapping. I was going to be consumed, I was going to be cut open, I was going to be chained. Demons were pulling at me, pulling at my clothes.

And then I was being rushed down a corridor. It reminded me of being rushed into the operating theatre. Was I going to be operated on again? Was I going to give birth again? What would be my fate? If only I could have got James to exit with me … Next time, I thought. I had failed in this life; I was supposed to get James to believe. Next time.

I could hear voices around me, they were the voices of my friends, friends from college, friends I'd grown up with. Were they with me? My eyes were open, but I could only see light and then darkness. I could hear the voice of Regina, a friend of mine who also had a son, who was saying, 'What's wrong with her? Let's get her in the room.'

The next moment, I was in a bright white room, wearing a hospital robe. The light was so bright, it made my eyes hurt. There was a metal gate latched around the room, tall sheet metal like an accordion. All that was in the space was a table and a chair. I tried moving on the bed, and I heard the sound of metal whooshing. What was that sound? Was it the wind? But we were in a room, there couldn't be wind in here.

I was still in restraints, thick belts around my wrists. A tall man with dreadlocks and glasses was smiling at me.

I saw his nametag, it said 'Nmandi, nurse'. The lights were bright, blaring in my eyes. I must be dead, I thought.

He was holding my hand. His grip was firm, steady. He looked so understanding, I felt at peace. He wasn't a demon, I knew this. He was on my side.

'Do you believe in God?' I asked him. 'Do you believe in heaven?'

He looked at me. 'Fifty–fifty,' he said. 'I haven't made up my mind, but I'm OK with that.'

'I'm a nurse here,' he said.

'Nurse, that's just a label that society has given you. That's just what's on your nametag. I see you,' I said.

And then I saw him, Nmandi, who spoke with his hands; he had the soul of my friend Regina in him. I could see he was also the author of *When Breath Becomes Air*, a man who helped those facing death feel less afraid. He was 'the nurse', the person who gave to his community, who held the hands of the dying and comforted those who mourned. I saw him in the fullest sense of the word.

And then I saw that if we were still in Hell, Nmandi must be the archangel Michael, coming to deliver us from Hell, from the demons.

He smiled gently at me and held my hand in the restraints.

'I'm going to take off your restraints,' he said, 'but I need you to behave and be calm. And then I can bring in your husband. Remember, you're dressed as a hospital patient, so he's going to see you as a patient. I won't let anyone come in the room unless you want them to. This room is a safe space.'

He unlatched my restraints gently. There were indents on my wrists from where I had struggled in them. He covered my legs with a blanket.

He left the room, and when he returned James was with him. James looked haggard and stood hesitantly in the corner.

'Does he know?' I asked Nmandi. And I meant whether James knew that we were in Hell.

'I know everything,' James said. He was crying. 'Please stop, Cat, please stop. You can stop now.'

What did he mean when he said he knew everything? Did he know that we were in Hell? Did he know that there were versions of his life where he was trapped in a hotel room for eternity? Had I ruined his ability to escape? Had I failed him? Perhaps he knew, which meant that he had been trying everything to keep us going, to help us escape Hell, to stop us living this loop, again and again. Was I not doing something correctly? I was Beatrice. What was I meant to do? *I surrender*, I thought.

'Now, I believe that you can get out of this. My shift is ending soon, and I'll have to go, so I want to help you get out of here,' Nmandi said. He paused. 'I believe that you and your husband can walk out of here, but you have to do it together, as a team.' He knitted his fingers together like a steeple. 'James, he's your anchor.'

'Anything that happens in this room, this is your safe space.' He established the rules for me. 'I need you to behave,' he said. 'No screaming, you have to act properly, or they will restrain you again. Remember, people are watching. Remember that you look like a patient.' I nodded, I tried to remember every word he said.

Nmandi left.

James was trying to smile.

'I'm sorry,' I said. I was truly sorry. Sorry for everything, sorry for not listening, for ruining James' escape plan. I should have trusted him. I should have surrendered.

'Don't be,' he said. 'I'm sorry for not listening to you. I'm sorry for not realising. I'm going to get you out of here, but you have to trust me.' Where was 'here'? Did he know we were talking about Hell? Did he know that we would have to descend?

'Where are we?' I asked carefully. It was a test.

'We're at the hospital, this is the emergency room area,' he said. Ah, I thought, so he still didn't know.

And in his face, I saw the desperation. 'I'm going to go talk to the nurses, but I need you to sleep. I'll be back. We'll go home.'

'I feel like we're being watched,' I said. I looked into the corners for the cameras. I thought I could hear the whir of them. I could hear loud noises from outside the room, voices and moans. 'We're being watched,' I said. And then I had a vision of us, reflected in a camera lens, zooming out from my perspective, and I could see us, James holding my hand, standing by the bed in front of the metal accordion walls, and me, lying on the bed, hands outstretched, the restraints next to me. I looked over at the door, there was a window there, with a blind. The blind was rolled up. Outside the window was bright light, and I saw a long table with people looking at screens and talking on phones. I could see Nmandi. He was talking with a demon, the eyes were slanted and dark, its features twisted. Nmandi was using his hands and gesturing at us. Then suddenly, there was a face in the window, the face of a demon peering in. He can't come in, I thought. This is a safe space.

'We probably are being watched, I think this is an observation room,' James said.

He kissed me. 'Why don't you sleep, and I'll go talk to the nurses and get us out of here. Just sleep.'

'Just sleep.' James' words resonated with me, as did my brother Teddy's, 'Just listen to James.' He stepped outside of the room, and he left the door open behind him.

I lay in the bed and tried to sleep, but I could hear the sounds of a hospital, every time I moved there was the sound of metal. I was in the maternity ward again, listening to the cries of babies, the sound of heartbeat monitors, of whispers. But where was Cato? He wasn't here. Above me, I could hear the sound of a camera's whir. *I have to look sane*, I thought. *I have to look sane.*

And then, as though a mist had lifted, I wasn't in Hell anymore, I was in a hospital room. I had clarity, I could see that there was a metal gate around the room, latched to the door. Every time I moved, the metal curtains made a sound like the opening and closing of a gate. I was in a hospital robe, I had indents around my wrists. My ankle was sore; I must have twisted it. I was lying in a hospital bed, there were bars and leather straps on the sides. I wondered if James would be able to check us out of the hospital, I wondered if this was going to affect my travel insurance. I thought of going home, home to London. Oh god, I thought. What a mess. I've made a mess. I needed to fix it. What would James' parents think? What would James feel? Where was Cato? I felt panicked. I needed to get out of here.

I wanted to stand up, run out the door, but I remembered Nmandi's words: 'You look like a patient, you need to behave.' I lay stiffly, but I couldn't sleep. My eyes wouldn't close. I got up to straighten the bed, the sheets were lopsided and dishevelled. Would I look insane if I was making the bed? Maybe I should just lie down until James comes back? I went to lie back down, but I couldn't lie still. I stood up again, adjusted the bed and lay back down. James had said this was an observation room.

What were they observing? Did I look insane? I stood up again; my ankle was throbbing. It hadn't been throbbing before. I started limping. Would they think I was insane for limping? Why was I limping? I straightened the bed sheets again.

I was looking ridiculous. I tried to lie back down and stay still, but my eyes stayed open, alert to the sounds of the hospital. I waited. I counted, but each time I got to ten, I needed to start over.

James had left the door open. Where was James?

There was an Asian man lying in a stretcher outside the room. He was haggard, his cheeks were hollowed, his face was thin; he was sitting in the stretcher and staring at me. He was cursing in Korean. 'Fuck, fuck.' A thought flashed in my mind. Was this James? Was James trying to talk to me? 'Why doesn't she sleep?' the man muttered in Korean. No, no it couldn't be James; we were in a hospital, that was another patient. Where was James? I stepped out of the door to look for him.

'You can't be out here,' a nurse said to me. 'You need to go back to your room.'

'I'm looking for my husband.'

She looked at me curiously. 'Where is he?'

'I'm not sure,' I said. 'He's working on checking us out. We live in London.'

'Mhmm,' she said. 'What's the date today?'

'I don't know.' I really didn't know the date. 'But I need to get back to my son, he's waiting for me.'

'Mhmm, how old is your son?' she asked.

'He was born 4th November 2017,' I said.

'So how old is he?'

'His 100-day celebration is this Saturday,' I said.

'Why don't you sleep?' she asked.

'I can't sleep,' I said. 'It reminds me too much of the hospital in London, the noises and the lights are keeping me awake.'

'You've been in a hospital before?' she asked.

I didn't understand the question. I had been in a hospital before, in the maternity ward. 'Yes?' I said hesitantly.

The nurse smiled at me, her eyes were sad. I guess I should have explained what I meant by a 100-day celebration. 'Go back to your room,' she said kindly. 'Just wait for your husband, he'll be back, he'll explain.' In the corner of my eye, I saw Nmandi shake his head at me and walk away.

Why did the nurse look at me so sadly, why did Nmandi leave? Was I still in Hell? Was this not actually a hospital? My thoughts started crowding my mind, and I thought back to the events, to my memories. Had I been right? How much time had passed? I had no sense of time. Was it no longer 2018? Was I actually in the maternity ward? Had I had a baby? Where was the operating theatre? Maybe I'd lost the baby? Cato? Was there no baby? The thoughts raced through my mind, one after another.

The nurse walked me to my room and closed the door. I could still hear the sounds from outside the door, I thought I heard someone laughing. It was a trick. I wasn't in a hospital, I was still in Hell. I must have failed.

I tried to lie in the bed, but instead I paced the room, limping. Where was James? How much time had passed? My hospital gown was wet in front. What was that? It was milk. I pressed my arms against my chest; my breasts ached. Where was Cato? He must be hungry, how long had it been since he'd fed? I needed to get to Cato.

I saw faces look worriedly into the room. Sometimes they were the faces of nurses, sometimes it was Nmandi, sometimes it was a demon.

'Fuck, fuck,' I heard the voice of the man muttering in Korean. 'Why doesn't she sleep?'

Maybe the man was James. Maybe James had already restarted, and because I wasn't restarting he had lived an entire lifetime and was now wasting away on a hospital bed. Why was James speaking in Korean? Was it a code? Was he trying to signal to me?

'Just surrender,' my mother-in-law had said. Is that what she'd meant? Why couldn't I sleep? Why did James keep saying I needed to sleep? I paced and paced, muttering to myself. I could see myself on a security screen, with my long hair and hospital gown, pacing barefoot in a small hospital room. On the bed I could see spots of blood.

In the nursing home in Virginia where I played violin, there was a woman who always asked to call her parents. 'Philadelphia,' she'd say. 'I want to call my mother in Philadelphia, she must be worried about me.'

'Later, when the phones are free,' the workers would say. They'd smile at each other knowingly, but after the fourth or fifth time, they would just ignore her.

There was a Korean woman named Na-hee, she reminded me of my grandmother. She spoke Korean with the same lilting satoori accent of the island people. She didn't speak English so I would sit and chat with her in Korean. Initially she didn't speak to me, but on my second visit, she greeted me like I was her daughter.

'Why's your hair so long now?' she asked. 'Why is it all wet from the rain?'

It hadn't been raining.

She showed me her doll, a broken thing with stringy hair and half-shut eyes.

I wasn't sure if she was as unwell as the others, it may have been the language barrier, but she followed the nurses' orders obediently and acted docile, like a child. However, the nurses told me that she had bitten another resident who'd tried to take her doll.

There was one visit when she was lucid.

'Let's go to my room,' she said. 'I can show you my view.' The room was shadowy, on the table was a comb of mother of pearl, a box of Korean snacks. She handed me one. 'You should eat more,' she said, and I smiled because she sounded just like my grandmother.

'We used to have a tree when I was a child. My brother loved it. My daughter loves to climb trees too.'

She stood by the window and her profile looked like my mother's, a strong nose and high cheekbones.

She turned to me, and I saw that she knew I was a stranger.

After that visit, she stopped speaking to me and would ignore me when I came in. Perhaps she didn't want to pretend anymore.

On my last visit, I sat with the woman who wanted to call her parents. She'd had a manicure, and her nails were a frosted coral pink. She was wearing pearls and a diamond pin. She had a ring on each finger. She held my hands in hers as though we'd known each other for years.

'Wake up, sit in a chair all day, and then sleep. It's no way to live. I'm used to going going going,' she said.

She was shaking her head, and I could tell that she was about to cry.

She was trying not to, but her eyes shone.

'Don't be sad,' I said.

'I know,' she said. 'I shouldn't be.'

When I left she smiled so hard her tears spilled over.

We are eating in the cafeteria. Will says, 'Jean, did you remember to get me a Valentine?'

She shakes her head at him, but winks.

Later, Jean brings out a cake she's bought for us. The mood is bright and the workers laugh as they set out the cake on the table. It's a sheet cake that says Happy Birthday with piped frosting roses in red and green. Jean cuts it into large squares. 'No arguing over the flowers,' she says.

We eat the cake with our hands, licking the spun sugar from our fingers.

'Happy Valentine's Day.' I remember my last Valentine's Day with James. I think of the words in his Valentine letter, 'I love you, boundlessly, unconditionally, steadily, I love you. Be mine. I'm already yours.'

And because I think I should, I write Cato a Valentine on a piece of pink construction paper.

Dear Cato, this is your first Valentine's Day. One day when you're older, I'll tell you about it. But you should just know for now – that I love you.

'Noona.' I heard my mother's voice. The door was opening.

'We are here, it's me, I drove seven hours to see you.' She sounded like she was crying.

My father stood beside her gruffly.

The door opened again.

'Noona. We are here, it's me, I drove seven hours to see you.'

James stood behind her, looking worriedly at me.

The door opened again and again. 'Noona. We are here, it's me, I drove seven hours to see you.' My mother said this each time, standing in a different place in the room. Sometimes crying, sometimes holding my hand, sometimes sounding angry.

What was this trick, I thought. A trick of the light. A reflecting trick. Which was my mother?

I lost track of the number of times they entered the room, hundreds of instances, shuffling in, shuffling out. I could hear my father's footsteps in boots. When I looked at their faces they were blurred, like someone had taken an eraser and smudged them out.

I screamed.

So I was in Hell. I decided that Hell was a computer simulation, a simulation of infinite possibilities, and now we'd come to this moment, and we were living this infinitely, trapped in an infinite loop. Was this my fate? I tried to make sense of the stories in my life, of the characters. I tried to find the patterns; I could figure this out. If we were caught in an infinite loop, then who was I? Who was James?

I thought of James' grandfather and how he had beamed at me the way James had during our first conversation. He'd lost his firstborn son, but he had so many grandchildren and great-grandchildren, he couldn't keep count of them. Had that been a version of James' life? Was this why his grandfather had been so happy to see me and Cato? Had that been James in another version of our lives?

Then who was I? James' grandfather had outlived three wives, was I the first wife? I never knew what happened to James' grandmother, the first wife, was she put in a hospital like me? Was that me?

The thoughts and memories flooded my mind and each brought a different answer that fit into a pattern with another. Was this what was happening? Was the world continuing on in an infinite pattern? We were all caught in this cycle, making the same mistakes we'd always made. Why had it taken me so long to see? If I was Beatrice, I must have failed, this was my punishment, the first wife, stuck in a hospital room, forgotten for eternity. I was Ariadne, trying to navigate the labyrinth, the Minotaur, but Theseus would leave me behind.

I remembered the story of a friend who found out that her father had a first wife who was in an insane asylum. He'd left her and remarried. He sent money back each year, and she stayed there, abandoned by her family, waiting, not knowing that time had passed. Was that me? Was I that wife? *I surrender*, I thought.

My parents were in the room again. My mother looked hollow, she was holding flowers in her hands.

My father's trench coat looked like a military general coat. Oh god, I thought. It's the Holocaust. It's beginning again. Outside the room, I could hear a building wave of voices. Souls of the deceased, I thought. I heard the sound of a metal gate closing, the walls were closing in. Oh god, I thought. We couldn't stop it. We couldn't stop it from happening again. Again and again.

'Are you in pain?' a man asked me. My breasts were leaking. Why?

Who was I? I knew this man. The name came to me. James. It was James.

Why was James looking at me with such concern, he looked like he was the one in pain.

Was I looking in a mirror? Was I James? Time seemed to reflect on itself, reflections of events happening again and again, but with slight variations. Perhaps I was on the other side of a mirror, looking into my reflection. Did that mean that everything I saw was just a reflection of what I was living? I started to imitate the world I saw around me; I was a reflection.

James was trying to spoon-feed me; he opened his mouth wide, gesturing at me to open mine. Wait. I wasn't James. That couldn't be right. Where was the baby? Was I the baby? Had I lost the baby? Was that why James was looking at me so gently?

'Do you have to use the bathroom?' he asked me.

I nodded at him, at my reflection in his eyes, I was looking at him looking at me looking at him. We were reflected there infinitely.

'I'm your husband,' James said. 'Say it after me.'

'I'm your husband,' I said. So I was James.

'No, say that I'm your husband.'

'You're my husband?'

'Yes, good.' He looked relieved. 'And you are …'

'I'm …' I paused. 'Cato?'

'No! No, you're Cat!' he said.

'Oh.'

He started to draw me a family tree with precise lines. I noticed casually that the words were blurred. I couldn't read.

How was I meant to exit this loop? I didn't understand how we could restart. I thought maybe we had to sleep. Sleep and wake up, destroy the old world and live again in the new. We had to exit somehow, we had to exit and wake up.

I tried to speak to my parents, to explain about the simulation, to let them know that we were in Hell. Perhaps they would understand me, because they'd been through this before, hadn't they? Wasn't that why my mother had always told me those stories? Wasn't that why my father had given me books on mythologies? Wasn't that why he had all his rules? I needed them to understand that we were in a trap, in an infinite loop, that we had failed this time, and we had to exit.

My mother had her hand on my forehead, she was smoothing my hair; it was like hers, long and dark as ink.

'Omma,' I said. 'James doesn't know, but we have to get him to sleep. I've been trying to sleep.'

'Yes,' she said. 'Please, please sleep.'

'I can't, I need James to sleep first.'

'James is sleeping right now, he's sleeping.'

'No, not just sleeping, real sleep, he has to restart. We have to restart this simulation.' I saw her face, it was blurring. It looked angry and uncertain. She didn't say anything, she kept patting my hair. Why wasn't she reacting? I felt anger, where was her sense of urgency?

'You have to believe me. Don't you believe your daughter?'
I started to cry.

She shook her head fiercely and blinked away tears.
'Stop it, you're not sounding like my daughter. My
daughter would never say these things.'

And then I knew, when I looked at her: she wasn't my
mother. Not my real mother. She was a distortion, a trick
of this mirrored world.

'I thought you were real, but I always knew you were a
devil,' I said.

I closed my eyes; I could trust no one.

The halls were crowded with people on gurneys, I could
hear the sounds of moans and screams. People would
appear only to be wheeled away moments later. Hell was
a busy place, I thought. My 'mother' would walk me to
the bathroom, I'd pass the station of doctors and nurses;
sometimes they looked like they belonged at a hospital,
other times their faces were distorted and scowling and
I saw them in their true form.

One of the patients on a stretcher was wearing the
clothes of a rabbi. 'I'm sorry,' I said to him. 'I'm sorry
about the Holocaust. I tried to tell my father, but he
wouldn't listen.' My 'mother' hushed me.

I'd often see Nmandi speaking to the people on the
stretchers. He would turn and smile gently at me through
the window in the door. Sometimes I'd wave frantically
at him, but his back would be turned and he wouldn't
wave back. *Yes, Michael, I've failed*, I'd think. What was he
thinking of me? Was he disappointed?

Outside the room were two guards. I learned that their
names were Lane and Fred, they were both big guys, but
they spoke to me gently and slowly. I knew who they
really were.

'Don't worry,' I said to Fred helpfully. 'In another life, you're a legend, a real hero. You even invent a grill.'

'Shush!' James hushed me.

To Lane, I made boxing motions. 'I hated every moment of training, but I thought to myself, suffer now and live the rest of your life as a champion.'

'Yeah, cool quote,' Lane said.

'You said it! In another life – you're a champion. So don't worry about this one.'

Lane smiled at me and shook his head.

Sometimes I saw Teddy, disguised as a nurse or a doctor. 'Teddy,' I'd yell. 'Help.' He was my foxhole buddy, perhaps he had always been, I thought of us together as children, whispering to each other as we waited for my father to stop his raging. We knew that we would eventually be safe, the moment would fast forward, like the VCR players that would fast forward the strip of tape.

'Teddy is in Seattle,' my false mother said. 'Noona, he is in Seattle. He's not here.' She handed me a mobile phone.

'Noona?' Teddy's voice sounded muffled. I knew we couldn't speak, we were being watched. I saw my mother's face look at me cautiously. I turned away from her.

'Noona, you're going to be OK.'

'Foxhole buddies,' I said. That was our code, our code to know that we knew what was really going on. We knew the truth.

'Yes, foxhole buddies,' he said. 'Don't worry.'

Maybe Teddy was watching, watching me from the ceiling. I looked up at the corner of the room where there was a blinking light. I tried to count the number of blinks. It was Teddy, he was telling me that it would all be OK. Teddy was watching from the ceiling. He would make sure this simulation would end. 'Just restart it,'

I whispered. I tried to blink in rhythm to the light, just restart.

I spoke to my father, the mathematician, to explain about the simulation.

'Infinity plus one,' I said to him. 'Because Teddy knows, he's a mathematician, it makes sense to him. We just needed to do it one time. Because this is a simulation.'

My father listened to me gravely. He waited until I had finished. He finally said, 'I can't promise you that we aren't in a simulation, but as far as I know, I promise we are not in a simulation. This is real.'

I sighed. He looked regretful, and I saw that there was a shadow of a man, a silhouette, one that was filled with loss. A contradiction. He held my hand, and I danced with him to a French song that I heard. We'd never danced at my wedding, or at least, in the wedding I remembered, but I knew that there must have been a version where we did.

'I went through the same thing you did, but I did it alone.' A nurse was braiding my hair. My hair was wet; I didn't remember her washing it. 'You're very lucky, your husband has been taking such good care of you. And your parents are here.' She looked at me. 'My husband left me.' She looked at me with red pupils, demon's eyes.

She pulled the comb through my hair, catching the snarls and carefully brushing them out. She started to braid, pulling one strand at a time, the way my mother used to when I was a child.

'You went through this too?' I started to cry. What was this place? Was this a hell for women like me? Were we all demons?

I tried to think of an escape plan, there must be a way out. I was becoming desperate. How was I meant to save James? How was I meant to stop this infinite loop?

'Catherine, I need you not to be scared, OK?' a demon said to me. 'I know you miss your baby.'

Was I Catherine?

I touched my hands to my stomach. My baby? Was there a baby? Where was the baby then? Maybe I'd lost it.

I could feel a jagged scar along the bottom of my stomach, what was this scar? I ran my fingers along the raised edges, it was a thick gash parallel to my hipbone. I tried to count, but I couldn't think of the words.

There was a buzzing in the room. It was the cameras again. They were rolling. I stared at the blinking red light. Blink. Pause. Sometimes it blinked, sometimes it paused. Outside the door, I heard the voices of my friends, my four closest friends, they were there, disguised as nurses. Why couldn't they come in?

'Come in,' I shouted. I called their names one by one. Why couldn't they come in? It must be because of my 'mother'.

I told her to let my friends in.

'No one is here,' she said. 'There is no one at the door.' She was lying to me. I could see their faces peering in.

'I promise you, your friends aren't here,' she said. I was too weary to get up from the bed.

'Will you promise to let them in next time? Can you promise that?'

'Yes,' she said. 'I promise.' She seemed to falter. Her face was blurred, she looked uncertain, like she was malfunctioning. Was that what was going on? I was trapped in a world of robots? Cylons?

I had a vision of the nurses, holding screwdrivers as they attached metal plates underneath my mother's face. Robots. *It must be robots, part of the simulation*, I thought. *Part of the trick.*

'Cat?' James came in with red flowers and containers of food. 'Cat, you need to eat, please.'

I looked at the food. It was human flesh.

'My mother made these for you,' he said. Poor James, he was being tricked.

I shook my head and started to throw the food on the floor, but he looked so sad that, even though it repulsed me, I stopped. He set up the table, I pretended not to notice he was serving flesh. I refused to touch it.

'Please eat,' he said. 'Please, just eat one thing.'

I shook my head.

He looked sadly at me. He looked haggard. How could I get him to realise we were in Hell? I wanted to exit, I wanted this to end, but I couldn't leave him behind, I needed him to know, I needed him to believe me.

'We have to sleep,' I said.

'Yes, please sleep,' he said.

'I need you to sleep with me.' I gestured to the bed, quickly, quickly before the guards came in and stopped him.

'No,' he said. 'Remember, Cat, we've talked about this before. It's against the rules.'

'There are no rules here,' I said. 'It's OK, the rules are in your head. I'm not going to leave you behind.' I spoke gently.

He shook his head. And so I failed again. I tried to remain calm, I would make him understand. I would.

*

Sometimes I heard the sounds of a baby crying. I could hear the sounds of a woman screaming. Who was screaming? Was that me? And then I heard the sound of a heartbeat. The heartbeat sounded like it was faltering. Was it mine? Was it James'? Was James dying? I heard the sound of a metal gate closing, opening, closing. There was a line connected to my wrist, I tugged at it.

Someone was piling blankets on the bed, pressing on top of my legs. I couldn't move, I felt paralysed in my body. I tried to scream, but there was no noise.

James brought more containers of food. There were biscuits, my favourite Girl Scout cookies, Oreos, a stack of crackers. There was juice, coconut water, a smoothie. He set them up carefully in a line, his on one side and the reverse mirror-image on mine. We sat across from each other on the floor, with our legs crossed.

'Let's have a tasting,' James said.

He took a sip of the juice. 'Follow me,' he said.

I imitated him. Perhaps we were in a mirror again.

'Refreshing!' he said.

'Refreshing!' I said.

I paused. James looked so thin.

'Why don't you eat?' I said to him.

James was crying. 'All I wanted was to give you a high-school date. You always said you wanted to go on a high-school date with me in my hometown. I'm sorry I never did that before.'

I looked at him with concern. 'It's OK,' I said. 'You always made me so happy.'

He hugged me, I hugged him close and tried to whisper the truth in his ear, but it only made him cry more.

*

I started to recognise the nurses, the same demons. They'd appear and disappear only to reappear again, wearing the same clothes, wearing the same expression. There was a nurse who never looked me in the eye. She'd glance at me with fear. I glared at her often, sometimes I bared my teeth. *Roar*, I thought. *Run, run*.

Sometimes I saw time fracture, a simulation of moments, James in duplicate, being tortured, living, waiting in a hospital room for eternity with me.

And then there was one time when I saw it: as he smiled at me, I saw a version where he left me behind at the hospital. He was dancing with a bride at another wedding, his own. There was a cloud of confetti and he was sobbing through his vows. I smiled. At least he would find happiness. I *was* the first wife. I saw that now.

I tried to explain to James that he needed to leave. 'I'm your first wife,' I said.

'No,' he said. 'You're my wife.' He pointed at the family tree.

'I know,' I said. 'But you will find another wife, and I need you to promise that you will. At least in this version.'

'This version?'

I nodded. I didn't want to scare him by letting him know how many versions there were where he was suffering for eternity.

I begged James for paper and a pen. He gave me a stack of paper and I started frantically writing down everything we were saying. If we were in a simulation, if we were being watched, Teddy would need this record to figure out what moment of time we were in. I wrote and wrote furiously. *Foxhole buddies. Bad storytelling, foxhole buddies, foxhole buddies, Cato you're killing your father.* I was trying to stop time, trying to pause the moment, what was the date, what was the time, how do you capture a moment in an infinite loop? I wrote until the pen ran out of ink. Frantic scribbles.

Sometimes music would play from the ceiling. James and I would dance. We danced to our wedding song, and I whirled with him and cried as he smiled, because with every turn, I was growing older, I was changing. I was Cato dancing with my father, I was a grandmother dancing with my grandson, I was James' first wife dancing to Ray Charles, I was his second wife dancing to a love song. James was trying to keep me in this moment, but it was impossible, we were caught infinitely. I held him close because even if I had him for a moment, a suspended moment, that would be enough.

I was still seeing patterns, still seeing connections. Every moment brought a new connection, a new pattern. The patterns, the connections I was seeing, there were too many of them and too many parallels. The stories and warnings my mother had told me were taking shape, I thought. Those stories had all been to prepare me for my fate, to give me strength for this moment. I saw that now. I had to be strong, I could not bend. Shim Chung and her blind father, was I going to drown in the ocean? Would I be reborn? Nong Gae dancing off the cliff, I was meant to be a sacrifice, to stop the oncoming tide.

I started to draw flowers, flowers on the paper, on the walls. I was Ophelia, dancing with flowers in my hair.

And then Cato was there, he was standing outside the door. He was an adult now, and I an old woman. When had that happened? Had my life passed, and I had forgotten it all? Was I in a nursing home? I looked at my hands, they were wrinkled, dry, my grandmother's hands. 'Cato,' I said. I wanted to see him, I wanted to see him before I forgot him again.

'He's not here,' my 'mother' said.

'I have to see him, he's standing outside, please, let him in.' I clutched at her shoulder, it felt frail in my arms. I could crush her, I could break this metal, then she would see, she would see. 'I have to see him, let me see him!' I shook her.

'No,' she said, I saw fear in her eyes. 'No, you can't open the door.' And then I sensed it, the moment was gone, Cato was gone, dead, disappeared. My chance had passed.

And for the first time, I wept. 'I'll never forgive you,' I said.

Outside the room, I heard the nurses talking about my husband. 'Her husband, first husband?' I heard Drew's footsteps outside in the hall. I saw him smiling, standing outside the door. Why was he here? Why was I trapped in this room? Why had they brought him? He wasn't my husband. Outside, I heard women screaming – who was he hurting? And then I realised who Drew was. He was every man who was cruel to women. We were the comfort women, he the Japanese soldiers. We were the wives, the ones who hid in the darkness, hiding behind concealer and false smiles.

I started to scream, I needed to exit this place, perhaps I was Alice in Wonderland, and I could shrink if I only ate the right thing. I started to chew on a piece of plastic I found that fitted on the bottom of a chair leg. Was I shrinking? Would I be able to hide?

I didn't know what I would do if Drew came in. I thought of all the ways I could kill him with what was in the room. A pen to the face, a cable cord around his neck, a shattering of the vase. I remembered the moment on the balcony, I hadn't had the will to fight then, but I did now. I knew now that I could not be prey.

Time split again, I was on the balcony, debating if I should leap. I was Leah, begging my son not to jump. I was Cato looking down from the balcony ledge. I could see the oceans below me, hands lifted up as if in prayer.

I thought of all the patterns in the universe, why had I never noticed them before? I'd been so blind. I was sensing something larger than myself. I was seeing the face of God. I was seeing the infinite.

I remember that when we were children, Teddy asked me what it would feel like to die. He was scared, he said.

I think he was seven and I was ten, I remember I couldn't imagine not being able to use two hands to count my age. I remember that I told him a child's version of heaven. And he smiled.

I remember that we were watching the hibiscus burn bright red in the fading light. We were looking out over the gravestones, the ones that lay empty. The black marble glinted midnight blue in the setting sun.

He reminded me of this a couple of years ago, when he came back from his trip around the world. He didn't believe anymore, he said. He'd seen all the beauty that nature had, he'd climbed mountains, spent days in solitude walking with only the wilderness around him. He'd lost his faith. No matter how hard he tried to find it.

He sounded regretful. He was still scared, he said. He had felt so alone.

In the ward, I have a glimpse of what Teddy meant. Days in solitude, without really talking, without really feeling. But I am waiting. I keep walking. To find the morning.

I think of Westbrook, my godfather. In the end, he had longed to die. He had sat by the window, his eyes closed, waiting for the night to come. His beloved wife had died first, of Alzheimer's. It had taken away her memories, her identity, and left a shell behind. Death was a friend, my godfather said, and he'd seen it often. It would be a place where soldiers were safe, where the young men he'd fought with would stand tall, would laugh, run free. It would be a place where his daughter would be, a child, always eleven. She died of cystic fibrosis, never able to fully take a breath. Death was the next adventure, he said.

It was finding morning.

I remember that James told me they were going to have to take me to another hospital. I was going to leave. A doctor stood by James; his arms were crossed. He was wearing silver spectacles. His voice was grave. 'She's been here for four days, and she hasn't slept,' he said to James, ignoring me. 'She doesn't seem to know who she is. She isn't getting better. Each time I've spoken to her, she is still confused.' What did he mean by four days? Each time he'd spoken to me? When had we spoken?

'I've never spoken to you,' I said.

The doctor didn't turn his head and acted as though he hadn't heard me.

But then maybe I had. Dr Jacobs. I tried to remember. I remembered being a child, drawing flowers with crayons, and a man nodding his head at me. His name had been Dr Jacobs ... But I hadn't been Catherine in that version. Or had I?

The world was a wash of colour; I could barely see anything. Where were my contacts? Where were my glasses? I didn't have my glasses. Why couldn't I see?

'Yes,' James said gently. 'It's because you were trying to chew on the glass.'

'But I can't see,' I said. Maybe this was my fate, to be blinded. Like my father. The world was just lights, blurred shapes of light and dark, and the people in it were figures that moved like coloured shadows. Was this how my father always saw the world?

Where was my engagement ring? My wedding ring? Was I not married in this version? My fingers were bare.

Lane told me that I was going to be going on a roller-coaster, he was strapping me onto a bed, my wrists were in restraints. I smiled at him, how sweet that he was trying to protect me from the truth. I knew the truth; I was going to be euthanised. I was leaving Hell, but I'd failed. I was going to be extinguished. I asked that he choose the fastest method. 'I want it to be quick,' I said.

'Let's not overthink it,' he said.

I always depend on the kindness of strangers, I thought. That sounded familiar.

Lane stepped into a vehicle, I saw that it was an ambulance, I saw the bright light of day, and I shaded my eyes, the sunlight was too bright. The air was crisp and clear, and I breathed it deeply into my lungs.

I started to sing as loud as I could, maybe Teddy would hear me. Maybe he could tell Cato about me, Cato would be too young to remember. I sang until the door closed behind me.

Time was still fracturing, I caught a glimpse of the world ending, again and again, apocalyptic. I saw a version where James was Ender, the one destined to close the universe. I saw Cato die, I saw Cato live, I saw him grow up without a mother, I saw him grow up with a stepmother, I saw Cato grow up to be James, I saw James as the youngest of three sons. I saw Cato's sons, I saw them die, and then be reborn again. I saw spaceships, I saw a Cylon war, I saw James fighting Cato, I saw floods, I saw Noah's ark, the fall of the gods, of Odin's son, I saw time bend.

And then.

*

I cannot see, I am holding my hands like binoculars to my face and calling them glasses.

I remember singing in French and pulling at my clothes.

I remember a gurney, and Lane holding my hands as I saw beasts pacing around me. What was happening? Was I in a pound? A zoo? An ape screams at me. An owl screeches. A panther stares at me from its perch.

I remember a light, a white room, plain. I hear a phone ringing. There are no windows, where is the light coming from? Was I going to be here for all eternity?

I hear the animals outside. 'No, no, you can't be here!' I hear shouting. I feel arms on me, hands on me, rough, and I'm being carried back into the white, back into the white room.

My legs are wet, is that urine? There is liquid on the floor. There are faces in the slot of the door, concerned ones. I see Drew's face, then my father's, then a demon's, then James', then my own.

I hear screaming, coming from within. Is that me? I'm screaming.

I hear James' voice shouting as though in a tunnel.

I am being put into a box, a box.

And then, and then, and then I wake up, with my hair tied in a strange way, and my breasts a network of knots.

I am in a room; the lights are bright, so bright I can hear them, a noise in my head.

There is the smell of chlorine and chemicals.

A woman is in the room with a mop. 'Breasts, breasts!' she shouts at me. I realise she means that I need to express. My breasts are swollen, I feel them, they are a mess of knots, red and sore to touch. Oh, I remember.

I was breastfeeding. I try to think about Cato, but the thought is pushed away.

The woman is slight with dark hair. She's wearing scrubs and rubber shoes.

She walks me outside of my room to the hallway, where she opens a door to a shower. She strips my hospital robe and gestures to me to express milk. I stare blankly at the shower head, there is no tap. 'Here, here,' she says. And jams a toothbrush into a divot by the shower. The water is ice cold.

She presses my breasts for me, motioning to me. 'Breasts!' she shouts. I mirror her.

'Change, change,' she says. She hands me a bra and a pair of underwear and maternity leggings. Those are my clothes, I think. There's a jumper which I recognise as my husband's. I wonder what he's wearing.

She drags a pair of large men's socks over my feet. I pad out to a bright hallway. I hear the sounds of phones, of the tapping on computer keyboards.

I hear a boy's voice, 'Hello, Cat.' He is walking along the hallway, he nods as he walks past. I wonder how he knows my name.

She walks me back to the room.

Before she leaves, she hands me a pair of glasses, and suddenly the world comes into focus.

I can see the room; it's plain and white concrete. There is a bed in the corner, but the sheets have been stripped. There is a window with bars at the top. There is a curtained partition, I open it and see a small bathroom, a toilet and a metal sink.

When I look at myself in the mirror, I don't recognise myself, I only see glasses.

I look around the room, at the single bed, at the shelving on the side. There are stacks of jumpers, leggings, underwear, cartoon socks. I touch them, one by one, slowly, they are my clothes.

I find a notebook under my pillow. It's grey with thick, pale paper. I recognise it as one of my husband's treasured ones. On the front page is his handwriting. Precise and neat. There's a list of names with phone numbers, and the date 9 February 2018 is written at the top. The year is underlined in thick ink.

So it's still 2018.

There is a purple marker on the shelf.

I tear out a page, and I write my truths.

I am alive, I write.

In Hong Kong, they believe that the spirit world is in the same realm as ours, only thinly separated, with spaces that overlap. The spirits, they watch us, from their realm. If life was cut off too quickly, they yearn to reach the living. Their presence can be felt in those moments – whether it's the wind or the call of the night, the spirits, they are here. And so, in this way, they are never separated from us.

When someone passed, you would stay at night in their home. You would light candles and prepare a large feast so that the spirits could visit and help guide the deceased's soul to the other realm. You wouldn't clean up the feast, you would leave it on the table, and before you left the room, you'd sprinkle the ground with white flour so that you could see the footsteps as they departed.

I loved that image of the footsteps of the spirit realm. It felt true to me, in a way. How many times had I felt the linger of a memory, the yearning of a spirit, of my grandmother. My grandmother passed away alone, on a quiet morning in the summer. Towards the end, she became like paper. She didn't have the energy to stand, she lay in bed, taking sips of water, listening to the sound of the ocean. I wonder if she thought of her island home, or if she remembered being a young girl and watching the war planes go by.

My grandmother started to forget, her memories of the past overtook the present. She cried for brothers we'd never heard of, she cried for babies unborn, she cried for her mother.

I hope the spirits heard her.

It is visiting hour. James comes with my father this time. James says that my mother wasn't sure if she should come. I think James also wants to spare her seeing me in a mental hospital.

It's the same number of guests again. Most of the cafeteria is empty. It's Emma, Mick and me. I see Emma embracing an older man and a young woman, it must be her father and sisters, I think. She's crying.

Mick is looking grave, the man who is with him stands slightly apart from Mick's wheelchair, like he doesn't want to be too close. I give James the Valentine for Cato. He blinks hard and puts it in his pocket.

My father is wearing his coat with the high collar. The one that I thought made him look like a general. His face is lined.

He looks hesitant; his eyes are owlish. He's not wearing his glasses, but he walks deliberately, footsteps clear against the linoleum floor.

I realise that in my nightmares, the footsteps I'd heard, the voice I'd heard in the halls, they weren't Drew's, they were his.

I meet his eyes, and I wonder if they will look at me with fear or curiosity, but they are just his eyes – dark oceans – and I realise they are the colour of Cato's eyes.

'Hi,' he says.

James is holding my hand, tracing the bones in my wrist.

'Hi, Appa,' I say.

He clears his throat, gruff, unsure. 'Look,' he says with a sudden smile. He takes out a fountain pen from his pocket and a piece of paper. He draws quickly, surely, his eyes almost touching the paper.

And I laugh.

I remember this drawing from my childhood. It's a silhouette of a man smoking a pipe, the silhouette is made of numbers. The pipe with a lazy curl of smoke is the number nine. His hat is the number three lying on its side.

'Number man,' I say.

'Yes, number man.' He looks shyly proud.

'You kept asking your father to draw this,' James says. 'You thought it had a hidden message.'

'I did?' I ask. I don't remember. I stare at the number man. An enigma.

We sit in silence. I don't know what to say, so with my other hand I pat my father's hand. James smiles at me. And I look at the two men sitting across from me, my past, my future.

When they leave, I stand to watch them go, James walks first, leading my father. My father shakes my hand, and he walks firmly, his footsteps echoing on the floor. He seems to linger, and he turns to me with an expression on his face that looks like regret.

I start to show people the photos that James gave me.

'Look,' I say to Nona. 'This is my son.'

I practise saying this, pointing at the baby in the photo.

'Ohhhhh.' She takes the photo from me. 'How precious.'

'How old is he?' she asks me.

How old is he … James told me over the phone that it was Cato's 100-day celebration yesterday. They had a small celebration at my in-laws' home. 'He's 100 days,' I say.

'You need to get better so you can go home to baby!' she says and nods fiercely at me. Shara is there too, she pats my shoulder and looks at me like she knows I don't recognise the baby in the photo.

'Don't worry, honey, you have a whole lifetime to get to know him.'

A whole lifetime? That seems inadequate. I've lived multiple lifetimes already. I want more than a lifetime. I want a lifetime of suspended moments.

In my notebook, I draw a woman with a baby in her arms. Her hair has a rainbow in it, a prism of colour. Her eyes are closed; she can't see the light. The baby is a curve in her arms, intertwined.

'You seem to be much better,' the doctor says. It's the one from before. It's been two days since we've spoken. She's still looking at the clock above my shoulder.

'I feel much more myself,' I say.

'Good, good,' she says.

'We're going to work on getting you home,' she says. 'You'll be able to leave tomorrow, we'll just have to prepare the paperwork.'

I feel like a window is opening.

'You'll get to go home to your husband, he's very worried about you.' She smiles at me.

My last night in the ward. I try to sleep, but I cannot. I am thinking of my lifetimes, my memories, those loops.

So now I know that when I am old, when I become like paper and start to forget, and my past becomes my present, I will cry for Teddy, a boy in corduroys who flies kites so high they touch the moon. I will cry for my father, a blind man, number man. I will cry for my mother, so beautiful, just thinking of her makes me ache. I will cry for James, my kind husband, who has conviction and a smile that could hold up the world, and I will call for Cato, my Cato, my son.

My grandmother used to tell me a story about one of her older brothers who lived on an island off the coast of South Korea, 'Dog Island', big enough for a village, and that was all. It is now an empty place. The younger generations left for the mainland, tired of the hard tides that surrounded it. My great-uncle, an old man, had been married for over forty years when he fell in love with a widow who sold sweet potatoes at the market.

Every night he would go out to meet her – the now disgraced woman – and his eighty-year-old father would chase after him with a stick and beat him and curse him all the way there.

My great-uncle would have let himself get beaten, I can picture this. He would have tried to move his shoulders so that each blow would fall more squarely on his back. Because then, at the end, his ultimate punishment would have been less. My grandmother said that my great-uncle would cry – both men would cry, the cursed one and the curser.

When my great-uncle lay dying he asked to see the woman. They wouldn't allow him; his wife and children stood guard over his bed – watched until he lost his last breath. There was a long funeral procession, his family carrying the box of ashes to let out at sea with the night tide. As my grandmother walked along the procession, she looked up and saw an old woman weeping in the mountains, running along the rocky path above.

'Following like a ghost in the traditional mourning clothes,' my grandmother said, 'a white dress.'

I can understand the beauty of this story – my weeping great-uncle, the ruined woman. What would her life be like after the ashes were put to sea? She'd been left alone, abandoned. They both knew that their ending would not be a happy one. This does not mean that my great-uncle was preparing himself for sorrow, hanging his head, waiting for the end – but that he expected it.

I think, though, that my great-uncle had a quiet hope, the hope of every great love story, that things will end happily ever after. It is that quiet hope that if they hurl themselves fast enough, they will come out on top. And then they realise. That that *is* the top. To reach that pinnacle of not caring about the end; to know that the end doesn't matter. This is the happiness of the ending, to have reached the point when the moment is enough, when to love is enough.

To fall fast, faster than gravity, faster than the ground can pull you back down, and find sky again, on the other side.

Tamyra gives me a reluctant hug. Her paperwork hasn't come through yet, which means she'll need to stay for another few days as it's a holiday weekend. She spends her time lying in bed, screaming because of her ear infection. Mick calls her a drama queen, but I hope the doctors will get her antibiotics.

'Thanks for teaching me Chinese Checkers,' Darren says. He's leaving today too.

'I can't believe you're leaving!' Emma wails. She asks that I promise to keep in touch, she writes her phone number in my notebook like we're leaving high school. *Stay cool*, I think.

Ali smiles at me before giving me a big hug. 'How much longer?' I ask him; that seems a safe question to ask. He shrugs. 'At least another month,' he says, and then he tries to laugh.

Christine tells me that I can start packing. I gather my clothing, James' jumpers, my notebook and scraps of coloured drawings, my beloved foam slippers. I offer to give Tamyra my toothpaste, thinking she'll be pleased, but she looks annoyed. 'I don't want *that*,' she says. 'You got any T-shirts?'

I shake my head, I feel sorry.

As I gather my things, I think of my grandparents and James' grandparents, the ones who fled their homes with their belongings on the backs of donkeys. Saying their farewells without knowing that it would be the last time, that there would be no reunion, only mystery and wondering. Lives interrupted.

They were suspended in the waiting, waiting desperately for the chance to meet again.

I think this is why Koreans are so obsessed with time and the past. They are yearning for something pure, for something they are never sure will happen again, and yet they wait, and they treasure the waiting, the yearning, because that is all they have.

And I take comfort that, even if I was not in it, there was a version of James' life where he would be happy, surrounded by so many grandchildren he couldn't keep track of them. And we would meet again, when he was 102, and I was with Cato, a newborn. And he would smile and hold my hand, and maybe he would, for a moment, recognise me.

'Your husband is here,' they say. 'He's here to take you home.'

I have a plastic bag with my possessions. I'm wearing boots. It's been so long since I've had shoes on that I shuffle in them. I am the first to leave the ward today, they tell me. I get to go first; my husband has been waiting since early this morning.

I walk the length of the hallway once more, past the glass enclosure, the nurses and doctors look up from their computers and phones and wave at me. Jeff gives me a hug. 'Take care of yourself,' he says.

Randy is waiting by the meds line. 'Bye,' he says. 'See you later.'

I wave.

I'm walking, one foot slowly in front of the other, following Christine.

She opens the door. I see James on the other side, he's teary-eyed. He reaches his arms out for me.

I step through the door. I don't glance behind me. This is my thousandth step, I think. I can finally breathe.

I take my first steps.

After my release, James took me to a hotel overlooking the Manhattan skyline.

'It's close to the hospital,' he said. It was unspoken, but the words hovered in the air. *Just in case.*

'We still have a few days before our flight back to London,' he said.

'We do?' I asked.

'Yes, our original flight,' he said. 'We're leaving in five days.'

I had spent a total of twelve days away from Cato, four days in the emergency room and eight days at the ward.

As we left the labyrinth of the brick building, I could sense the air changing, becoming sharper, clearer. And as we exited through the thick doors, each step felt magical – the cars, roads, people, it was familiar and yet new.

James held my hand as he drove, and we arrived at the hotel with a lobby of copper and brass. I listened to our footsteps echoing on the tiles, to the people leaving, smiling and chatting. Did they know that they were free? Where were they going, I wondered.

The lift had mirrored walls, and I looked at my reflection unsteadily. My hair was falling down over my shoulders, tangled and unruly. Was I marked? Did I look the same? I felt caught in my reflection. James looked at me worriedly. 'Let's go,' he said.

'I think you'll like the room,' he said. 'I tried to set it up so that you'll be comfortable.'

The room was a wide suite, with tall windows. We could see the skyline rising above the river.

James closed the door, and we sat on the floor, holding hands, staring at one another. He looked thin, and his hair was falling over his eyes.

'What do you want to do?' He sounded uncertain, and his voice shook.

'I just want to be here,' I said. I listened to the sound of rain on the windows, the sounds of the silent hotel. 'What do you want to do when we go back home?' I asked.

James smiled, a hesitant smile. 'Home, that sounds nice.'

Home was an idea, the future was an idea. I couldn't think of the past, there were too many lifetimes to remember. The future felt safe, I was with James, it would be OK. We talked carefully about the future, small details, I told him that I'd missed hot drinks, and he laughed as he made me a cup of tea. My hands curled around the porcelain mug, I'd missed the feel of porcelain in my hands.

We didn't talk about what had happened the past few days. We avoided it. It hung in the air heavily. It was like waking up from a dream.

I showed James my foam slippers proudly – 'These were my favourite possession' – but he looked sad and upset, so I set them aside.

I lay in the hotel bed and revelled in the soft sheets, the feel of the pillow cool against my cheek.

We feasted on sushi, spicy Korean stew, oysters, ice cream, mochi. I had lost fifteen pounds since being admitted. James set up the food in a single line on the coffee table, like he had in the hospital. We sat across from one another like reflections.

'It's like a mirror,' I said. And James looked at me sharply.

'Cato is at my parents' house,' James said. I hadn't asked where Cato was, but James pretended that he hadn't noticed.

I learned that my parents were at my in-laws' house as well, taking care of Cato. They had cancelled the 100-day celebration party and had a quiet gathering at home. James showed me the photos of Cato surrounded by pale blue streamers and a small plate of rice cakes, and I stared at them without recognition.

On the first night, there was a heavy snowfall. We walked outside in the quiet white evening, holding a red umbrella. We watched our feet sink deeply into the snow, leaving footprints of white. The highways were still, and the only sound was of the snow falling. I thought of the ward and tried to imagine seeing the snow from the window in the television room. I was free now. I breathed the air deeply, taking in the cold, taking in the fullness of the snow. And I felt, for the first time in a long time, peace.

My parents brought Cato to the hotel on the second day. My mother looked thinner, more fragile. Her eyes met mine, and I could see a sliver of hurt there that I didn't know if I could repair. My father stood gruffly in his coat and nodded. He was holding Cato, who was curled in his arms. His eyes looked at me, unexpectant.

As I thought, I didn't recognise Cato. He looked like a stranger. I searched myself for some emotion, but I couldn't find any.

'Don't you want to hold him?' my mother asked.

I forced myself to nod.

He felt heavy, like an unfamiliar weight. I tried to remember how to hold him, but he was much bigger than I remembered. He didn't seem comfortable. He didn't look at my face; he just looked over my shoulder, struggling back and forth. He didn't look like the photos, his face was different, and his eyes that used to be devils' eyes looked at me innocently. His hair looked strange. 'His hair started falling out,' James said.

I looked at Cato. My son, I reminded myself. And I felt nothing. We were separate beings, truly separated. It was like he had been cut from me, again. I looked into the distance, outside the window, where I saw the outlines of New York City and the fog from the river.

My father quietly took him back from me, and I saw my parents look at each other with concern.

I sat on the bed and stared out the window, while my father paced with Cato in his arms. Cato started to cry, and my mother handed my father a bottle.

'Oh,' James said apologetically. 'He's on a bottle now, but he seems to like it.'

I shrugged. *All that struggle*, I thought dully.

'How are you?' my mother asked. She touched my hand gently. She looked like she was about to cry. 'Did you eat well?' I smiled at the typical Korean greeting.

I nodded. 'I'm fine,' I said.

My parents left quietly, promising to visit the next day. 'Get some rest,' they said. They didn't meet my eyes when they left.

James and I walked along the harbourfront, the city shone like glass, glittering bright against the metal of the sky. We walked side by side, hands clasped, James feeling steady and grounded against me.

It felt like we were existing separately from the rest of the world, except that sometimes James had to be on the phone to the insurance companies to discuss our flight and my medical bills. 'I don't want you to worry about this,' he said. And he'd carefully shut the door behind him and speak so that I couldn't hear.

He told me later that he'd been on the phone with the insurance companies for hours, trying to find out if my hospital stay would be covered. 'We need to get back to the UK,' James said. 'I miss the NHS.'

My eyesight was still blurry and I couldn't read. I showed James my notebook.

'Do you want to read it?' I asked.

'Later,' he said. 'I'll read it later, when we get back home.'

The days passed by slowly. We'd wake and walk along the harbourfront, trudging through the snow. We'd pick up breakfast and eat on the floor of the hotel room, talking over hot cups of coffee and buttered bagels. My parents would come with Cato and stay for a while. I'd hold Cato sometimes; he didn't seem to be getting used to me, but I'd touch his face and the softness of his hair.

It was a Tuesday morning when we checked out of the hotel, and our flight was that evening. I had to wonder what the hotel staff thought – my parents walking in and out with a baby, James and I taking long walks around the harbour – but the receptionist looked bored, perhaps our actions didn't seem out of the ordinary. I thought I caught a glimpse of a demon's eyes from her, and my breath caught in my throat.

'We're going to go to my parents' house,' James said. 'Is that all right?'

'Yes,' I said. I wanted to see it before I left.

As we pulled into the neighbourhood subdivision, it didn't feel menacing, just familiar, it was just a house. James' father was waiting outside for our car. He embraced me, laughing as we slipped in the snow.

I took a deep breath as we walked up to the door. James' mother embraced me fiercely, she was crying. She stared at me and asked if I was all right. I nodded.

'Have you been eating well?' she asked. I smiled.

My mother-in-law had prepared tables of food. 'I wasn't sure what you'd want to eat,' she said. She seemed shy, and sometimes she had trouble meeting my eyes.

My parents were upstairs, and they came down with Cato. My mother hugged me, while my father patted me awkwardly on the shoulder. 'We're going to leave,' my mother said. They were preparing for the drive home. 'Take care of yourself,' she said. It was an abrupt goodbye, and I stood by the glass door to wave as they drove away.

I stayed on the couch, quietly sitting with a cup of tea, while Cato slept on a mattress next to me. James' parents were talking softly to each other in the kitchen, while James was upstairs on the phone with the insurance companies again. I felt numb. I couldn't feel relief or joy; I was out, I was free, I should be feeling light, but instead I felt weighted and dull, like I was in a tank of water.

James' parents drove us to the airport, and when we left for the departures terminal, I turned to see them, waving slowly, gravely at us, worry imprinted on their faces.

On the flight back to London, I looked out the window, to the clouds, to the curve of moon. The beginning of the trip seemed so long ago. Time no longer felt linear to me, I had too many repeating moments, too many gaps.

Back in London, I let James take care of Cato, while I lay in bed and read my notebook, looked over the scraps of paper, the frenzied notes, the pages of lions, unicorns and bears coloured in marker. My memories felt sharp, raised like a scar. I still had to take my medication, three pills that looked small in my palm. An antipsychotic that made my brain feel numb and my hands shake, a pill that countered the side effects of the antipsychotic, and a sedative that helped me sleep at night.

Eventually James and I would talk about those days. James would tell me that he knew something was wrong when I asked to leave his parents' house, but he wasn't sure what it was. He told me that Teddy also realised something was wrong during our phone call. I learned that he and James decided that they would try to get me to calm down and to sleep. However, by the time James took me to the hospital, I was manic, stripping my clothes and screaming in the emergency waiting room. James told me the hardest moment was watching me as I was fighting with the nurses while they clamped me in restraints.

James' memory of those days in the hospital was that I was frantic, in constant motion, talking one moment about Greek and Norse gods and screaming the next. Sometimes he was able to distract me by asking me about the past or by playing question games, but sometimes he wasn't able to, and I'd address the ceiling and talk so quickly I'd bite my tongue. The only way that he could get me to eat was to sit in front of me and have me imitate him. He said that I was obsessed with the date written on the number board above my bed. Eventually, he said, they erased it.

Sometimes I referred to myself as Beatrice, as James, as Cato. Sometimes I thought I was a child and drew scribbled pictures like a pre-schooler, and other times I thought I was an old woman. He said there were times I seemed lucid, and that those moments were the hardest: he could see the terror and confusion in my eyes. He said that he could get me to smile by dancing or reminiscing about the past. But no matter what he did, he couldn't get me to sleep. It was on the third day that James called my parents to come up from Virginia.

James said the conversation was confused. 'You have to come now,' he'd said. Had there been an accident? No. Was I unwell? Yes, and no, not physically.

'I don't understand,' my mother had said.

'It's an emergency,' James had said. 'It's an emergency. Cat is really sick. Mentally sick.'

They'd driven up to New Jersey and gone straight to the hospital. When they came in, I didn't recognise them. I stayed lying in bed and chattered to the ceiling, making shadow animals with my hands. They stayed with me while James went home to sleep.

Teddy said that he couldn't come, he had too many things going on in Seattle. James' eyes narrowed when he told me this. I learned that they had argued about it.

'My being there won't help her get better,' Teddy had said. He was calm, measured. 'This is temporary, she is going to get better.'

James couldn't understand how he had seemed so unconcerned, so unfazed.

'He knows me,' I said. I understood, it wouldn't have helped to have Teddy there, and I didn't know how to explain to James that Teddy had always been there, a voice on the phone, talking me calmly through each nightmare.

James said that I had refused to talk to my mother, we would argue. She had to spend most of the time standing in the hallway; her presence agitated me. However, my father would listen to my raving quietly. He would sit by my bedside and hold my hand, nodding and saying he understood. He would ask questions about Dante's *Inferno* and the Greek mythologies.

James told me that the decision was made by the hospital team that I needed to be admitted to an involuntary ward.

He told me that when they transferred me, I was singing loudly in French. The song I was singing was Édith Piaf's 'Non, je ne regrette rien'. He had played it for my parents that night, and my father wept.

I learned from James that the animal pound I thought I was in when I reached my most manic state was actually the high-security area of the psych ward, and the animals were the security guards. James had watched as I screamed and fought and was restrained by the guards. He was shouting too, but they kicked him out of the room.

He said that as he sat in the waiting room, listening to my screams, a man asked him if he believed in God.

James said, 'No.'

The man said, 'Well, now is the time to start. I will say a prayer for your wife.'

I like to think that that man was a guardian.

James said that while I was in the room, fighting and screaming, I stripped off my clothes and urinated on the floor. I was eventually sedated, and for the first time in days I was able to sleep.

He told me that the happiest moment for him was when Teddy called to tell him that I'd called. That I'd sounded like myself. He told me that he had made two other visits, ones that I don't remember. He said that I'd seemed agitated, fidgety and had spent most of the time drawing pictures on pieces of paper. He said that one of the workers had braided my hair, and it had made him feel reassured, that I was being taken care of.

James and I talked about those days until it didn't frighten us anymore. My sense of what was real and not real was blurred, but slowly I was able to reconstruct what was reality and what was my psychosis.

Once my eyesight became better, I read obsessively about post-partum psychosis. I joined a forum of women who had experienced it. I read about the fear, the isolation.

I learned that for most women, post-partum psychosis occurs a day or two after the birth. It was unusual for it to occur when the baby was already a few months old. My official diagnosis was stress-induced post-partum psychosis. While the reasons for post-partum psychosis aren't fully understood, the symptoms are usually similar – paranoia, racing thoughts, delusions, an inability to sleep. I heard from women who had been convinced their baby was a demon or thought their baby was going to catch fire. There was a woman who had forgotten she'd had a baby, and she wept every time she discovered her C-section scar, and another who was convinced that her baby was not her own. One thing that was shared by all these women was a feeling of separation from their child, and I could sense from the forums that there was a deep sense of shame from the women who had been unwell.

I read news stories, sensationalised ones, and my breath caught when I read of a woman who jumped off a bridge with her newborn baby.

I learned that if we'd been in the UK, I would have been admitted to a mother–baby unit, and not as a regular psych patient as I was in the US. I learned that the medication I'd been prescribed, haloperidol, would have been unusual in the UK, as it is considered to be extreme. The treatment in the UK is focused on keeping mother and baby as close to one another as possible, in order to minimise emotional separation; in the UK, I would not have been separated from Cato. When I read this, I felt angry. The separation had been unnecessary, the rules felt so trivial and arbitrary, and they had such an impact on our lives. I had come back a stranger, and the distance I felt from Cato wasn't something I could grieve; it went beyond loss. It was a severance, a removal that was complete.

I learned that we had been lucky to avoid any further separation. The state had threatened to call child services because I was potentially unfit to care for Cato. James had been worried that we wouldn't have been able to come home, lost in a bureaucratic nightmare.

A part of me was also angry when I found out that the ostensible reason given for why we cancelled the 100-day celebration was my 'exhaustion'. Did the family really believe that? I wondered. But it wasn't for me to contradict.

'People wouldn't understand,' my mother and mother-in-law both said to me on separate occasions. I understood. And so I kept quiet and tried to smile when people asked about my exhaustion, and whether I'd had enough rest.

In London, I was assigned a team to oversee my recovery. They were called the Mental Health Crisis Team. James and I met with a perinatal psychiatrist, who listened quietly to what had happened. I remember that I told her the story in the past tense, as though it was now behind us. We were optimistic, buoyant even. I asked her about coming off my medication, but she told me that we needed to wait. I think she knew that there was still more to come.

A few weeks after our meeting, I fell into a deep depression. It is a common occurrence after post-partum psychosis and taking haloperidol antipsychotic medication. It seemed instantaneous, like the descent of darkness under an ocean, immediate and complete, without any memory of the light that had been there before. I felt stripped of any life force. I didn't have the strength to lift a spoon; when I sat up, my entire body ached. I had never known anything like this, I couldn't even form a smile, it hurt my face too much.

I spent my time in bed. Each day stretched out in moments, while I stared at the blankness of the ceiling. I spent the hours trying to will myself to breathe, trying to will myself to stand up, and not being able to.

I felt like I was at the edge of something, something that would swallow me whole. I could sense a vastness I didn't understand, sometimes I could feel its quiet approach, and I thought I was going to be lost, and I didn't know what to do. In those moments I would close my eyes and count and try to stay.

The crisis team visited me every morning at my flat to check in. I forced myself to get out of bed when I heard the bell ring. Sometimes I'd be able to brush my hair, smooth my clothes, most days I couldn't. I sat very still, a presence on a chair. I was aware I had a body, but I couldn't be sure that I existed. 'How are you feeling today?' they'd ask me.

I would try to form words, to find the breath behind my voice, but most of the time I would not be able to answer. They would look at my face and say, 'You will get better,' and they would smile. 'This will pass.' And I tried to believe them, in the promise in their smiles.

They told me to make lists, goals for each day, things to do. There were pages of lists in my shaky handwriting. Each task seemed insurmountable. 'Get out of bed. Make a cup of tea. Play the piano. Make a phone call. Hug Cato.'

Their visits each morning only lasted a few minutes. But those minutes were precious, a promise of light in what felt like an abyss. I felt grateful for each task they gave me, and I would mark them off my list, my hands shaking as I tried to hold a pen. There were some days when I felt the promise of light for a longer moment, but then it would be gone, and I would return to looking at the vastness. I felt like I was slowly drowning. I was reaching for emotion, but there was only a silent desperation, and it felt absolute and unending.

As I lay in bed, I often wondered about the other residents in the ward. I'd think of Tamyra, had she had her baby? I wondered about Emma, and what happened to her after we had all left her behind. Did Ali finally get released? And Will, was he homeless? Was he on the streets? And Darren with the gentle voice, would he be OK? I wondered about all of their stories, interrupted, I'd only caught a glimpse of their lives.

My mother came to London to visit every few months. While I lay in bed, she would stroke my hair, which had grown long and brittle, and worry over the marks on my skin. She would massage my legs and arms the way Korean grandmothers do, trying to stimulate blood flow – *it'll be good for you*, she said. She told me stories and scolded me like the old times, chattering as she cooked my favourite dishes and tried to coax me into eating. I knew that I'd caused her pain, but I had a deeper understanding of her love.

I had a sense that after my psychosis, she had let me go. 'Spend time with James,' she'd say. And she'd smile as I would finally sit up from bed to walk with James to the park.

'It's hard,' she said when I couldn't swallow a spoonful of the soup she'd made for me. 'It's hard not to be able to make your child happy.' And she'd look at me with an expression that I didn't fully understand. 'When you were a baby, when you were a child, all you needed was me to make you happy.' *You will understand* – it was unspoken, but the words were there. Love flows down.

My father did not visit; he faded back into absence. However, I learned from James that my father had come with him to every meeting at the ward; that my father would play Satie on the piano in the lobby, and they'd listen to the notes echo in the hall. James told me that as they waited for the doctors, they would talk about mathematics, about Kentucky, about my childhood. 'I wasn't kind to her,' my father had said.

James said that my father knew I was back to normal on their last visit to the ward because I didn't talk to him. It's when he drew number man for me. Perhaps he knew that we were back to the way things were.

When I heard that, I didn't know what to feel. I knew that I felt some of the regret I had seen on his face as he left the ward that day. I thought about talking to him, but I didn't know what I would say. Words seemed inadequate. And perhaps he already knew.

Teddy would call me every day on the phone to check in. He spoke to me gently. Sometimes he'd ask after Cato, but mostly he would ask after me. I'd told him what my father had said to James, and Teddy had given a short laugh of disbelief. 'I know,' I'd said.

Thinking of Teddy made me feel wistful; like I wasn't sure if I was thinking of a version of a boy who no longer existed. But I don't think that's true, he will always be my foxhole buddy.

And James, he was patient with me as I waited to come back to myself. He would walk slowly with me, hand in hand, through the park under the fading sun. And I would try to remember what it felt like to feel something, anything.

I don't know if psychosis brought us closer together, I hope that it did. What I do know is that it changed something profoundly in James. The eternal optimist that I knew and loved now has a darkness in him, something that casts a deep shadow. I was upset when he packed an emergency hospital bag in case I had another 'episode'. I watched him lay out supplies on the bed: a phone charger, spare bottles for Cato. It made me nervous, I said. It was unnecessary. But he shook his head, he wouldn't be caught off guard again. He had been shaken, his certainty, his sense of control had been lost.

James said there was a time while we were at the hospital when he thought maybe I wouldn't get better, and that this was going to be our reality. And he didn't know what to do, except to wait.

He'd been sitting in the hallway outside my hospital room, trying to pause, to understand what was happening, when Lane had put a hand on his shoulder. He told James he'd been watching us dance. He was just getting over a break-up, he said in a confiding tone, and James laughed despite himself. Love problems.

'It's nice you're here,' Lane had said. 'Most people leave. They can't handle it.'

Sometimes I would think about that pull I had, the thought that I had to restart, to 'exit'. It would frighten me and leave me feeling hollow, like I was standing over a precipice or looking at the expanse of the ocean. It was love that saved me. I was sure of that. My love for James, my refusal to leave him behind. I'd thought that was my sacrifice, but in actuality, it was what had saved me, from myself.

My depression would last for several months, and each day I struggled to come back, to the surface, to myself. My interaction with Cato was a few minutes each day at most. I would hold him in the mornings while James got ready to go to work. Holding Cato felt wrong, unnatural, even painful. I'd count the seconds until I could get away with giving him back.

It was May when I was able to move my body without effort. I no longer felt like I was underwater. I was becoming myself again.

I could remember glimmers of emotion, like joy or hope, but I couldn't remember what it felt like to love Cato. He was still distant from me. I had thought that in becoming myself, I would find my son too. I thought of my love for Cato as being buried within me; surely being a mother was something that had been imprinted on me, it would be waiting for me. But when I looked at Cato, he could have been anyone's baby. The curve of his hands, the lines of his face, they were unfamiliar. He no longer belonged to me.

I didn't understand how our relationship could be so fragile. Those months of carrying him in my body, the hours when he'd slept in my arms, that fierce possessiveness, how could it be erased. The only way I could understand it was that it was an intention. Perhaps I had sent him away from me, an instinct to protect him from a mother who couldn't be trusted. Perhaps, I thought, it was an act of love.

The thought didn't comfort me. When I looked at Cato, it was a reminder of what I'd lost, that whatever connection there had been was gone and, it seemed, would never come back. I thought I should want to mourn, but I didn't feel any longing for him either.

It made me feel like a hollow shell. I would stare at Cato, and he would stare back at me, at his mother, a mother who couldn't smile or hug him. I wondered if he could sense it, this stranger who had taken his mother's place.

So I went through the motions. I reminded myself to reach for him, to smooth his hair when it fell across his face, to stroke his cheek. I practised smiling at him, thinking this is what a mother would do. I wondered if there was a way to build love and, if there was, did that mean it was manufactured, less real.

I took my medication faithfully. I counted the colourful pills in my palm each week, lining them up in the pill box James had ordered for me. I would stay on the antipsychotic and antidepressant for a year. I watched my body change from the medication, until it no longer felt like my own. The doctors adjusted the dosages, and I felt relieved when they started the process of taking me off them completely.

And to Cato, I asked him to wait. To wait for me to come back. And while I waited, I looked for joy in the moments with him. I listened to his laughter, I clapped when he learned to take his first steps, and I held his hand when it was outstretched for mine. I looked for the suspended moments, the ones that I needed to capture.

And then one day, an ordinary day, as I was holding him, I remembered him. His smile, the feel of his breath against my arm, the warmth of sun against our cheeks, the weight of his body against my own. And I was a mother again.

Acknowledgements

I want to thank my agent, Sophie Lambert, for her wisdom and steady guidance. Thank you for taking a chance on me and for being the most amazing champion for this book. Thank you for making this dream come true.

Thank you to Molly Atlas for her brilliance and for shepherding this book in the US. Thank you to Katie Greenstreet, I'm so lucky to have you on my side. Thank you to Kate Burton, Alexander Cochran, Matilda Ayris and to everyone at C&W agency. Thank you to Kelly Oden and the team at ICM.

I am so grateful to my wonderful editors, Angelique Tran Van Sang and Caroline Zancan. Thank you for your support and guidance through this process. I'm so inspired by your intelligence and passion, and I really can't believe how lucky I am. Thank you to Alexa von Hirschberg for your faith in this book. Many thanks to Kerry Cullen and the teams at Holt and Bloomsbury for their care.

Thank you to my early readers – Emma Bailey, an inspirational human woman generous with her genius, Betty Ho for reading countless drafts and giving incisive advice, Emma Claire Sweeney for being a guiding hand as always. Thank you also to Ileen Park, Arzu Tahsin, Jonathan Ruppin, Georgina Simmonds.

I am indebted to our friends who supported us during my recovery – Marta Vergnano, Regina Aberin Tran, Susan Zheng, Ariane Ling, Aileen Sun, Janet Lau, Anita Lin, Irwin Tran, Enrico Berardo. I cherish you all. Thank you to Jane della Pena for the help you gave to our family. Special thanks to Tom Ward and his boeuf bourgignon (it made it in the book somehow!)

I am so thankful to Jonny Geller for your mentorship and counsel. Thank you to my pod, Lucy Morris, Lucia Walker, Abbie Greaves, Jess Whitlum-Cooper, and of course, EB2 for your thoughtfulness and for sending brightness when I needed it most.

I would like to thank the many health care professionals who took care of us – that this is something you do each day for anyone who passes your doors is awe-inspiring. Thank you to the teams at the hospital and medical center, every kind word and caring action made a lasting impression. Special thanks to Nmandi for being such a light and to Lane for your kindness.

I am very grateful to Dr. Sarah Taha and the Mental Health Crisis Team for being a lifeline, thank you to Dr. Anthony Jolley, Dr. Anna Solly, and Sharon Judd and the FIRST Mental Health Team for your expertise and care.

I would like to thank Dr. Hong for so generously giving us your expertise.

I am thankful to the writing teachers I've had over the years for sharing their expertise and love of the craft. I've never forgotten the lessons and encouragement you gave me – Judy Turner, Melanie Cameron, Olivia Birdsall, Pat Hoy, Bonnie Friedman.

Thank you to the Choi family, Paul, Sara, Bill, Lori, and especially Abonim and Omonim for your love and support. Thank you to my family, Omma, Appa, and Teddy, for being my foundation and for helping me come back to myself. Thank you also to Omma for being the one to show me how to tell a story.

Finally, to James, you were and are my anchor, thank you for being there, for dancing with me even in the hospital, and for always making me feel safe in your love. Thank you to you and Cato for your patience and love, this has been our journey.